DID YOU KNOW THAT . . .

- The average American eats 10% less but weighs 14% more than his counterpart at the turn of the century.

- Physical, mental and emotional circumstances can determine and change metabolic rate.

- Muscle used regularly by someone who exercises vigorously 3 or 4 times a week is relatively active at *all* times.

- A high capacity for oxygen protects against diseases of the heart, lungs and blood vessels . . . but dieting lowers the body's use of oxygen dramatically.

- Overeating speeds up your metabolic rate.

- One secret of fat loss is *duration,* not intensity of exercise. Walking for long distances rather than running for a couple of miles is the most effective way to reduce.

"*Dieting Makes You Fat* is fascinating."
—*Library Journal*

"A real boost for those ready to abandon the traditional fad-diet merry-go-round."
—*Kirkus Reviews*

D0423667

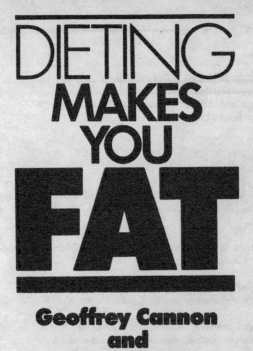

DIETING MAKES YOU FAT

**Geoffrey Cannon
and
Hetty Einzig**

PUBLISHED BY POCKET BOOKS NEW YORK

Originally published in Great Britain in 1983 by
Century Publishing Co. Ltd.
First revised edition published in Great Britain in 1984 by
Sphere Books Ltd.

POCKET BOOKS, a division of Simon & Schuster, Inc.
1230 Avenue of the Americas, New York, N.Y. 10020

Published by arrangement with Simon & Schuster, Inc.
Library of Congress Catalog Card Number: 85-2451

ISBN: 0-671-62530-6

First Pocket Books printing March 1987

10 9 8 7 6 5 4 3 2 1

POCKET and colophon are registered trademarks
of Simon & Schuster, Inc.

Printed in the U.S.A.

In memory of
Surgeon-Captain T. L. Cleave
1906–1983

ACKNOWLEDGMENTS

Professor Per-Olof Åstrand, Sir Douglas Black, Dr. Denis Burkitt, Dr. Kenneth Cooper, Dr. Denis Craddock, Professor John Durnin, Dr. Katherine Elliott, Dr. Elizabeth Ferris, Dr. John Garrow, Dr. Kenneth Heaton, Dr. Hugh Trowell, Caroline Walker and Professor Peter Wood read this book, or pertinent sections of it, before its publication, and gave us encouragement and advice which we have incorporated.

Dr. Keith Ball, Professor Michael Berger, Dr. Jeffrey Bland, Dr. David Booth, Ben Cannon, Will Chapman, Dr. Michael Church, Helen Cleave, Surgeon-Captain Hugh Cleave, Surgeon-Commander Brian Cliff, Dr. Michael Colgan, Professor Michael Crawford, Dr. Alan Maryon Davis, Mike Down, Wendy Doyle, Professor Richard Edwards, Susan Einzig, Malcolm Emery, Dr. Oliver Gillie, Barbara Griggs, Professor William Haskell, Professor Mark Hegsted, Victoria Huxley, Professor Philip James, Professor Harry Keen, Leslie Kenton, William Laing, Dr. Derrick Lonsdale, John McCarthy, Alistair Mackie, Mary Mackintosh, Tom McNab, Dr. Michael Marmot, Professor J. N. Morris, David Nabarro, Dr. Eric Newsholme, Professor Ralph Paffenbarger, Vic Ramsey, Dr. John Rivers, Christopher Robbins, Dr. David Ryde, Professor Bengt Saltin, Lillian Schofield, Professor Aubrey Sheiham, Professor Jeremiah Stamler, Dr. Andrew Strigner, Professor Albert Stunkard, Professor Paul Thompson, Colin Tudge, Dr. Richard Turner, Professor Roy Walford, Professor Arvid Wretlind, Brian Wright, Celia Wright, Arthur Wynn, Margaret Wynn, Dr. John Yudkin and

Professor John Yudkin gave us advice or guidance on particular aspects of the book.

We owe thanks to everyone who helped us. The responsibility for the views in the book is of course ours. Once again, we will be glad to hear from any reader who wishes to comment on any points we make.

The climate that has allowed us to prepare the book has been created by friends, colleagues, and workers in the field, whom we would also like to acknowledge.

At the *Sunday Times* in London, John Lovesey and Norman Harris have championed the cause of health and fitness for all; and Don Berry has supported our ideas. At *Running* magazine, Sylvester Stein, Alison Turnbull and especially Andy Etchells have supported the projects that turned some of the thinking behind the book into living experience. Cardiologists Dr. Robin Hedworth-Whitty and Dr. Peter Williams, together with physiologists Ted Charlesworth and Kevin Sykes, and Dick Hubbard, Rita Rowe and Ian Jamieson supported these projects. At the Body Workshop, Barbara Dale, Catherine Mackwood and Esme Newton-Dunn have shared their experience and enthusiasm.

For the London 1982/50 project, special thanks are due to Will Chapman, Jim Cockburn, Rosemary Evison, John Goody, Michael Jacob, Hilda Nyman, Rosemary Tempest and John Walker; to Terry Bennett, Peter Bird, Don Clark, Steven Downes, James Kelly, Ken Walker and Stan Weber; and above all to Simon Morris. For the Fun Runner '82 project, as well as those already mentioned, special thanks are due to Bill Brown, James Godber, Dr. Barrie Gunter, Mick Rankin, Bernie Tuck and Wendy Wood; and to Allan Appleton, Vic Burrowes, Tim Burton, Vivienne Coady, Bill East, Jane Heywood, Michael Innes, Rodney Lewis, Teresa Malinowska, Liz Parry, Bobbie Randall, John Routledge and Eileen Ward. For the Getting in Shape project, special thanks are due to Professor David Denison, Malcolm Emery, Dr. Bob Green, Jane Howarth, Tom McNab, Dr. Andy Peacock, Bev Risman and the staff at the National Heart and Chest Hospital and the West London Institute; and above all to Will Chapman. Everyone connected with these projects is to be thanked, some three times over.

Personal support was given by Kathy Crilley, Corinne McLuhan, Teri McLuhan, Charlotte Parry-Crooke and Rosalind Schwartz, and by our families.

Sir Douglas Black, President of the Royal College of Physicians of London, has been the presiding genius of three reports, on Medical Aspects of Dietary Fibre, Inequalities in Health, and Obesity, all of which have influenced us.

Inspiration and encouragement has also been given by Graham Alexander, Dr. June Burger, Dr. Michael Cohen, Helen Davis, Bob Donovan, John Falkiner, Tim Gallwey, John Gravelle, Bob Kriegel, Ian McGarry, Michael Murphy, John Poppy, John Ridgway, Mark Shapiro, Paul Spangler, Leslie Watson and Sir John Whitmore, all of whom have contributed some spirit to the book.

Professor Marshall McLuhan became a dear friend and a teacher who encouraged the knowledge that progress often requires looking a paradox in the eye. This book is the poorer for having been written after his death.

Deborah Rogers, our agent, and Gail Rebuck, our British publisher, together with Susan Lamb, Sarah Wallace and Anthony Cheetham, had the courage of our conviction. Penny Phipps and Deborah Brain put the show on the road. We owe special thanks to them.

ADDITIONAL NOTE

As the much longer list of acknowledgments in this new edition indicates, we have been given the most generous encouragement, criticism and advice from authorities in America, Britain and Europe who, with us, are convinced that plenty of whole food and plenty of fresh air are not only the reliable treatment for overweight, but also the means to a full, happy and long life. Thanks to this support we have been able to incorporate into this edition much new research and new thought, together with other work we had overlooked.

Above all we owe thanks to the hundreds of readers who have written to us, giving accounts of their own experiences and asking for advice. While we have not written a cookbook or a series of exercise programs, we have, in response to readers, written new passages designed as practical guides to nutrition and exercise. So, this edition is indeed "revised, updated, and expanded."

CONTENTS

PREFACE

This is not a diet book. It is a book about dieting. It is also a guide to energy, food, fitness and health.

By "diet" and "dieting" we are not referring to the type of food that people eat because of their cultural habits or religious and ethical beliefs (as in "vegetarian diet"). When we say that dieting makes you fat, we are talking about the diet regimens followed by people who wish to lose weight (as in "calorie-controlled diet"). We are using the word "diet" in this latter sense.

This book is not for people who are very fat, who, indeed, may be suffering from a metabolic disorder and need special hospital treatment. A woman of normal height weighing, say, 250 pounds or more may need to be semistarved and kept under medical supervision in order to regain her health. We are writing for people who are not ill; for the scores of millions of people in the West who are fatter than they want to be, who have tried dieting, who have found that dieting does not work and who want to know why, and what to do.

We do not recommend the use of drugs as a way to lose weight. It is our conviction, shared by doctors who have supported us in the preparation of this book, that now is the time for people to take responsibility for their own health and to avoid drugs whenever possible. Able-bodied people do not need drugs to lose weight, and any drug devised to suppress appetite or to speed up metabolism is liable to be dangerous.

The research for this book was the joint responsibility of the two authors. The book was written largely by Geoffrey Cannon, and the "I" throughout the book is therefore his except in Chapters 6 and 7, which were written from a woman's view by Hetty Einzig.

INTRODUCTION

Overweight and obesity are the most serious public health problem in the United States, Britain and other Western countries. And the problem is getting worse. In January 1983 the Royal College of Physicians of London published a report on obesity. Commenting on surveys of men and women in the last fifty years, the report states: "There now seems little doubt that there is a general trend for both men and women to become heavier and presumably fatter, this change being particularly evident in young adults."

This British report confirmed similar findings of scientists in the United States and other Western countries. Americans, too, are getting fatter. In 1981, it was officially estimated in Britain that about a quarter of men and women in their twenties and just under half the population over forty are carrying excess weight. The figures in America, according to the U.S. Society of Actuaries, show that over half the population above the age of thirty is overweight or obese. If you assume that these figures merely demonstrate that we are eating more, they will not surprise you. But we are eating less. Government statistics show that since 1960 we have consumed a steadily decreasing amount of food and drink, continuing a century-old trend.

It is generally assumed that fat people are greedy and that they not only eat too much but also eat more than lean people. How could it be otherwise? But in 1982, Alison Paul, a leading nutritionist, reported that children and teenagers are eating less than their parents, are consuming anything from 300 to 500 calories a day less than World Health Organization recommendations, yet are more likely to be overweight than underweight. Professor Harry Keen of Guy's

Hospital in London conducted a survey of 3,000 adults which showed that those who ate most had least body fat. And in 1984, Professor Peter Wood of Stanford University in California, reporting on studies carried out in Britain, the United States and other Western countries, confirmed to me that "generally speaking, fatter people eat less than thinner people."

DIETS SLOW YOU DOWN

These puzzling facts are not well known, and I have yet to read them in any diet book. This is because they suggest what millions of dieters have found out for themselves: that diets do not work.

An older generation used to say that fat people were unlucky, because they had "something wrong with their glands." A more sophisticated version used the word "genes" rather than "glands." A theory which has recently become fashionable is that fat people are stuck with a "set-point" programmed to make them fat. This is a variation of an older idea that fat people are burdened with a "low metabolism." From the point of view of the fat person who wants to be thin, all these theories are bad news. They all imply that some people are born to be thin, others born to be fat, and that there is not much anybody can do about it.

But this notion is contradicted by the example of people living in settled rural communities untouched by Western influence, who often live to a ripe old age and eat well without getting overweight, let alone obese. Moreover, before the Industrial Revolution few people in Western countries, other than the rich, got fat. The theory that all of a sudden fatness became inherited is absurd.

Books on dieting tell you to concentrate on reducing the amount of energy you take in from food. And most will tell you that while exercise is good for you, it won't make much difference to your weight. Stay sedentary but go on a diet, is the message. Yet the studies cited above have shown that although they eat much more food, active people are leaner and lighter than sedentary people.

EXERCISE SPEEDS YOU UP

When we talk of "metabolism" or, more correctly, "metabolic rate," we are referring to the speed at which the body uses energy. The diet books assume that while different people have different metabolic rates, every individual has a fixed rate—that the metabolic rate we are born with is the one we are stuck with.

The exciting news is that metabolic rate is not static: it is dynamic. As scientists have known for more than fifty years, dieting slows the body down and certain types of exercise speed it up: well-established facts that, if published in diet books, would damage their sales. Within wide limits we can choose the speed at which we want our bodies to work, and we can develop a faster metabolic rate by the right kind of exercise. The body gradually adapts to endurance exercise by losing fat and gaining lean tissue. This training effect allows us to eat more while losing fat, because working muscle is very much more metabolically active than body fat.

It is only in the past few years, as a result of the running and aerobics boom, that millions of people have transformed themselves from overweight dieters to leaner, lighter, fit and healthy people, who exercise a lot and eat a lot too.

GOOD FOOD—THE RECIPE FOR HEALTH

The main single cause of the diseases that most of us in the Western world suffer and die from is the food we eat, combined with inactivity. Western food lacks nourishment because most of it is highly processed. And one of the main processed foods we eat—sugar—is unique in containing no nourishment whatever.

It isn't enough to avoid highly processed food. The sedentary life that most people in Western countries lead is unnatural. The choice for sedentary people is gloomy. Either they stay light in weight by continual semistarvation, depriving themselves of essential nourishment; or else they consume enough food and get fat because their bodies cannot use the energy that comes with the nourishment. Either way they are liable to suffer ill health.

The sure way to good health is through fitness. Regular vigorous exercise gives the body the capacity for food for which it was designed. Regular exercise brings with it the freedom to eat as much as you like. Active people can best enjoy their lives by eating whole food, full of nourishment.

The best medicine is plenty of fresh air and plenty of good food: a remedy many family physicians once recommended, but now overshadowed by the propaganda of big business, technology, drugs and surgery. As Hetty Einzig and I did the research for this book, we came to realize that much more often than not, dieting creates the conditions it is meant to cure. By slowing you down, dieting makes you fat.

It is our conviction that dieting is not only self-defeating but also a means whereby tens of millions of men, and at least twice as many women, are prevented from enjoying their own lives.

You can change your life only when you know that you are able to make the change. The helplessness dieters feel about their weight and shape often undermines their lives. This book may encourage you to take your life back into your own hands.

Confessions of a Dieter

A man or woman may live and work and maintain bodily equilibrium on either a higher or lower energy level. One essential question is, what level is most advantageous? The answer to this must be sought not only in metabolism experiments and dietary studies, but also in broader observations regarding bodily and mental efficiency and general health, strength and welfare.

—W. O. Atwater and F. G. Benedict
*Bulletin of the U.S. Department
of Agriculture, 1902*

Quality. You know what it is, yet you don't know what it is. But that's self-contradictory. But some things *are* better than others, that is, they have more quality. But when you try to say what the quality is, apart from the things that have it, it all goes poof! . . . Obviously some things are better than others, but what's the *betterness?*

—Robert C. Pirsig
Zen and the Art of Motorcycle Maintenance

3

MEMOIRS OF A FAILED DIETER

I found a slip of paper recently, folded into an old wallet. It read:

> 2 eggs boiled or poached
> 4 ounces of lean meat *or* boiled fish
> 1 slice bread
> 2 water biscuits
> ½ ounce butter (level dessert spoon)
> ½ ounce sugar (level dessert spoon)
> 1 ounce milk (two coffees white)
> 2 ounces hard cheese
>
> In any amount:
>> water (3 pints at least)
>> tea, coffee
>> pickles, dry spices
>> peppers (only "fruit" allowed)
>> lemon
>> chemical sweeteners
>> green salad (only vegetables allowed)
>
> All else forbidden, including:
>> butter + ½ ounce
>> sugar + ½ ounce
>> alcohol
>> fruit, fruit juice

Dieting connoisseurs will recognize this daily regime as a version of the high-protein diets set out in *The Doctor's Quick Weight Loss Diet* by Dr. Irwin Stillman and in *The Complete Scarsdale Medical Diet* by the late Dr. Herman Tarnower. My version was sterner about fruit and vegetables, and cheated a bit with the butter and sugar.

A lot of people believe the Stillman and Tarnower diet regimes: to date, their books have sold a total of 20 million copies worldwide. "I'm convinced that the Quick Weight Loss Diet is the finest and best for most people who should take off excess weight," wrote Dr. Stillman in 1967. "No diet has ever been so spontaneously and unanimously acclaimed as this one," wrote Dr. Tarnower in 1978. He went further: "I urge you to get started now on this diet. Every day that you delay and keep or increase that extra poundage is impairing your appearance and your health, and is endangering and shortening your life. Overweight is a kind of death for almost everyone, slow for some, quicker for others." Fervent words.

I first tried the high-protein diet in 1970. It worked. My weight came down by 41 pounds, from 190 to 149 pounds, in twelve weeks. I had reached and passed my target.

Between 1970 and 1974, despite two intermediate purges each of 12 pounds, I had regained over 30 pounds. In 1974 I went on the high-protein diet again. This time I followed the word of Stillman more faithfully, adding fruit, vegetables, tuna with all the oil drained, diet soda, and mustard to the regime. I cut out sugar and butter but allowed myself one sin—a glass of wine. It worked again. From 180 pounds, my weight came down by 10 pounds in two weeks; by 20 pounds in four weeks; after six weeks I had lost 25 pounds. Then, after nine weeks, by a dizzying and ecstatic effort of will, I broke the 150-pound barrier; and I held steady at 146 pounds between weeks twelve and sixteen.

Like psychiatrists and schoolteachers, diet doctors often have a way of suggesting that if all goes according to plan the credit is theirs, whereas if you fail the fault is yours. I believed them. By New Year's Day 1976, I had regained 32 pounds. At midnight I made a New Year's resolution and, for a week, followed the regime set down in Dr. Allan Cott's *The Ultimate Diet* and in Shirley Ross' *The Super Diet*. I fasted. Not a pea. Just water. Well, a small sin: milk in coffee.

After three days, I found, as the books had predicted, that hunger faded, and I felt clean, light-headed and sharpened. More to the point, after ten days I had lost 15 pounds, finishing up at 163 pounds. But by the end of April, I had regained 16 pounds.

I was good at dieting. I could always win a lose-weight contest. My first epic diet was of the "sensible" type recommended by Professor John Yudkin in his book *This Slimming Business* and, more recently, by the Consumers' Association of Great Britain in *Which? Way to Slim:* low carbohydrates; cut down, or out, bread, pasta, cereals, confectionery, cakes, biscuits, potatoes and alcohol. "A low-carbohydrate diet is good for general health, not only for slimming," says the *Which?* guide. This worked too: I lost over 20 pounds, which I regained in two years. I was, as I recall, this failure that led me to try most other diets, once. Nevertheless, regarding bread and potatoes, as well as sweets, as bad, on two or three other occasions I cut out carbohydrates and lost 7 to 10 pounds in two or three weeks.

LOSE WEIGHT ON POTATOES

My biggest weight loss was on a "single-food" diet. These diets, often touted as fun, do not count calories but restrict the dieter to one or a few foods. The more ingenious versions stipulate a food normally seen as a treat, which, in due course, you come to hate. Examples are the grapefruit diet, the milk and banana diet and the ice-cream diet. Single-food diets are usually sold along with some mumbo-jumbo about the special qualities of the food to be eaten.

Judy Mazel's Beverly Hills Diet is a skillfully marketed version of the single-food diet. It restricts the dieter to exotic fruits (mango, papaya, with pineapple) for days at a time. Since the average-size woman would have to eat 8 pounds of mangoes a day to supply her normal energy requirement, it is hardly surprising that the Beverly Hills Diet works.

Any single-food diet will work, whatever the food. In a classic experiment—of rather more nutritional significance than Ms. Mazel's diet—twenty-three young Irishmen from Galway, organized by Dr. Denis Burkitt, volunteered to eat ten large potatoes, baked in their skins, every day for three months. Most of them lost weight, for the potatoes gave them about 1250 calories a day, less energy than the male body normally needs for its maintenance. No one yet has become rich and famous propagating this Irish diet, which is surprising in a way, since the volunteers were told that they could eat anything they liked every day, after they had eaten the potatoes. As it was, they found they had little room left for pork chops or profiteroles.

My own version of the single-food diet was oranges—with the occasional tomato. The principle of this regime was that I liked oranges and tomatoes; and I still do, surprisingly enough. In three months in 1967 I dropped over 40 pounds, from 185 pounds to 144 pounds. I celebrated by buying a suit, which fit for two days and then hung in my wardrobe, unworn, for fifteen years, a memento of two days in my life when I was thin.

Between 1964 and 1976 I lost about 200 pounds. If all my diets had worked, on New Year's Day 1976 I would have weighed minus 20 pounds. The records I kept were full of notes like "Halfway there!" and then "Failed" and "Failed again." Most of my life consisted of backsliding from diets. Was it the spoon of sugar, the glass of wine? I supposed that between diet regimes I "let go"; I felt bound to agree with Professor Yudkin:

> The upshot is that if you take too much food, containing too much fat and carbohydrate (or to a much lesser extent too much protein), you will be piling up an excess which you will store as fat. . . . In the end, it is food, and only food, that makes you overweight.

I read this as meaning that I was greedy. Gaining weight was a visible sign of an inward weakness; of a general failure as a person. If I didn't diet I feared that I would balloon up to look like the Michelin Man. This horrid fantasy drove me to further diet regimes.

Dieting is a private matter. Like "dirty" books, diet books are not read in public places, because in both cases people are ashamed to reveal how they fall short of what is expected of them and what they want to expect of themselves.

OH! MISERY!

I tried psychology. On another slip of paper I wrote "Being Fat Means":

Clothes don't fit. Good clothes hang, wasted, in the wardrobe. I pretend drab and baggy clothes are best.

I get tired, especially at weekends. I loll around listlessly, and may even sleep in the afternoon.

Food is obsessive. I eat, feel bloated, and then feel hungry again. I look for eating companions.

Embarrassment. In clothes shops, on a beach, with friends, playing cricket, seeing people after a gap of time.

Depression. At lack of self-control, at evidence of middle age, at knowledge of impaired health.

Gaining weight and being fat appeared to be my most intractable personal problem. I hated myself physically and despised my ineffectiveness. I didn't shape up. When I crossed the 180-pound line, self-respect or self-hatred would motivate me, and I'd go on another diet regime. Dieting was my dirty little secret, but actually I was not alone.

In 1978 the British consumer magazine *Which?* surveyed 1001 dieters, 788 women and 213 men. The main single reason given for failure as a dieter was "lack of willpower and determination." "I know how to lose weight. I know I can lose weight. I lack the willpower to keep at it for what amounts to a lifetime, because whenever I give up on the program I put it on again," said one respondent. And another: "I am very good at losing weight but once the loss slows down I give up and tend to put it all back on again." As for me, two couplets by Theodore Roethke come to mind:

> *Self-contemplation is a curse*
> *That makes an old confusion worse.*
> *He who himself begins to loathe*
> *Grows sick in flesh and spirit both.*

But what to do? I ate, I wanted food, I grew fat. Food, hunger, appetite, my body, were my enemies.

TOO MUCH ENERGY IN, TOO LITTLE OUT

Diet books usually say that fat people either eat too much or take too little exercise. That seems common sense. So, I thought, maybe my vice was not greed, but sloth. Most diet books do not, however, forecast a slim future for the fat exerciser. "It is extremely difficult to lose significant weight by exercise," says Dr. Tarnower. "A half hour of energetic bicycling, for instance, uses up 200 to 280 calories, which you put right back on by eating an iced cupcake." And Dr. Stillman: "Even walking at moderate speed for a full hour uses only about 200 calories; no amount of exercising will reduce you if you overeat."

Professor Yudkin looks kindly upon exercise but says, nevertheless, that "to dispose of a single cheese sandwich you would have to play squash for an hour. And to dispose of a good business lunch, you would have to play squash for eight hours." At a press conference held by the Obesity Research Foundation in London in August 1982, Derek Miller of Queen Elizabeth College repeated the claim made in diet books that to get rid of the energy content of a hearty meal it would be necessary to walk up and down Ben Nevis, Britain's highest mountain.

Clearly, from what I had read, exercise could do little for me. The British Code of Advertising Practice on slimming aids confirmed this view:

> A diet is the only practicable self-treatment for achieving a reduction in excess fat. . . . Claims, whether direct or indirect, that weight loss can be achieved by any other means are not acceptable.

The message was clear. Fat people eat too much. Slim people do not hike up mountains after dinner, nor do they get on their bikes after eating a cupcake. The damage was done by greed, not sloth. The partner in sin was the calorie.

CALORIE COUNTING

I dropped the thought of exercise and turned to the diet books which claimed that by self-denial and using their regime, I could lose 10 pounds or more a week. I was a dieting expert. I believed the diet books worked. If after I stopped the diet I regained the weight I had lost, I was sure the fault was mine. I was a backslider. I was greedy.

What should I weigh? My ideal related to the tables of "desirable body weight for men" published in books and magazines, and pasted on weighing machines. These tables, devised by an American, Louis Dublin, for the Metropolitan Life Insurance Company, categorized people into arbitrary large-, medium-, and small-frame sizes.

According to the tables, my "desirable" body weight at slightly over 5 feet 11½ inches, wearing indoor clothing, is supposed to fall somewhere within the following figures:

	Frame		
Height	Small (lbs.)	Medium (lbs.)	Large (lbs.)
5'11"	144–154	150–165	159–179
6'	148–158	154–170	164–184

These "desirable weights" varied from a little less than my heaviest weight ever to my lightest: a range of 40 pounds. The range for a woman of average height is 25 pounds. I decided privately that "large frame" was polite for "fat" and that the tables were nonsense. Nevertheless, they retained their fascination. While I had no idea of what the weight of my own body should be, I had a dream: I aspired to the bottom of the "small-frame" scale. I wanted to reduce myself to a statistic.

How much should I eat? Diet books rely on textbooks that list recommended energy intake. A calorie as defined by a standard work of reference is:

A unit in which energy is measured. Technically, a calorie is the amount of heat necessary to raise the temperature of a gram of water one degree Centigrade. Food energy is measured in kilocalories.

(A kilocalorie is 1000 calories. But most people, nutritionists included, refer to a kilocalorie simply as a calorie.) The U.S. Government recommends that the energy intake of a "standard" man of 154 pounds and 5 feet 10 inches tall who engages in "light activity" should be:

Age	Daily calorie intake
19–22	2500–3300
23–50	2300–3100
51–75	2000–2800
76+	1650–2450

"Light activity" is defined as "sleep or lie down for eight hours a day, sit for seven hours, stand for five, walk for two, and spend two hours a day in light physical activity," which summed me up well enough, in those days. "For adults, it is believed that an 800-calorie range covers most individuals," says one textbook. And to take the most extreme range, the energy requirement of the "standard" seventy-six-year-old woman 5 feet 4 inches tall and weighing 120 pounds is 1200 calories a day at the lowest end of the scale, while the top end of the scale for a nineteen- to twenty-two-year-old woman is 2500 calories a day.

The bigger you are, the more energy you need. And the older you are, the less energy you need, because people tend to slow down as they get older.

Diet books tell you to cut down your energy intake from food to 1500 calories a day or less. Audrey Eyton, in *The F-Plan Diet,* says: "Allow yourself 1500 calories daily if you are male, of at least medium height, and more than 7 pounds overweight. . . . Allow yourself 1000 calories daily if you are female and less than 14 pounds overweight."

Dr. Tarnower says, "The Scarsdale Medical Diet averages 1000 calories or less a day." Dr. Stillman is very stern. "You may falsify a calorie total on paper, but your body adds correctly and will turn into fat any extra calories that you omit by fake mathematics." At one point he recommends a lettuce, lean meat and hard-boiled egg diet totaling 354 calories a day. Another Stillman diet, for the fainter-hearted, is the "Six-Meals-a-Day Nibbler Diet." Of this he says, "Whereas 900 to 1000 calories is the usual number allowed on a calorie-counting diet the nibbler diet allows you 1200 to 1800 calories a day." This caloric cornucopia is against Dr. Stillman's nature. "For desirable quick weight loss," he goes on, "start with 900 to 1200 calories daily and then you may increase after you've learned control."

Diet doctors tend to be stern. Dr. Arnold Fox devised the Beverly Hills Medical Diet (BHMD: it has nothing to do with Judy Mazel's Beverly Hills Diet). "Lose ten pounds in fourteen days! Enjoy potatoes, pasta and other forbidden foods," promises the front cover. But when Dr. Fox comes to define what he calls "freedom with responsibility" he says, "You are permitted to mix different recipes and to redesign the menus according to your personal preferences—provided you don't exceed the 1200 calorie limit." And he goes on: "Consult the BHMD calorie chart to determine the calorie count of each recipe."

"The fewer calories you consume, the more quickly you will lose weight—within limits," writes Professor Yudkin, and "A daily 1000 calories is normally recommended as the safe low-calorie limit." Whether diet books favor fiber (Eyton), protein (Stillman, Tarnower) or carbohydrate (Fox) or oppose carbohydrate (Yudkin), the story is the same: lose weight by cutting calories, usually to 1000–1500 a day.

Dieters feel that their fat is their fault and that they are fat because they eat too much. Dieting is fueled by guilt and self-disgust. Many dieters feel that the most conspicuous and inescapable evidence of their general failure to manage themselves and their world is their fat. Fat people believe that they are unfit and unhealthy. Hatred of being fat, and fear of becoming fat, are demoralizing and disturbing to the point, for many dieters, of affecting their mental well-being. I know: I was there. I was alienated from my body; it was out of control. Cyril Connolly wrote, "Imprisoned in every fat man, a thin one is wildly signaling to be let out." The thin being has been taken over, surrounded, in the most literal way, by the alien, fat being.

But what to do? I dieted, I lost weight, I regained the weight, I grew fat, I was my own enemy.

COULD IT BE GREED?

Something that vaguely puzzled me at the time was that I didn't think I was eating all that much. "Self-deceit!" say the diet doctors. An acquaintance of mine, a specialist physician with a busy private practice of fat patients who want to be thin, regards them as naughty children who need discipline: firm instructions, an ordered regime. Otherwise, he tells me, they'll always cheat. The usual fable of the health farm is of the delinquent fatties who at dead of night lure their fellows in obesity to a gastronomic orgy at the local five-star restaurant.

Did I raid the icebox more often than other people? Were my portions larger, my meals bigger? Was I addicted to snacks? Diet books even include stories of people who go on sleep-walking binges. Could that be me? I watched friends and colleagues as we ate. They shoveled it in; they were not fat. I ate, feelings of self-disgust alternating with feelings of "To hell with it, I'm fat." Was I really eating more than they were? Did they raid the icebox? Did they buy candy bars on the way home? These are questions you don't ask.

Some people do, indeed, eat compulsively, and thereby become obese. I was sure that the average fat person was a big eater—and that gargantuan appetite led to obesity. Why else should people get fat? For a Briton, the images are of two kings, Henry VIII and Edward VII, the one throwing gnawed haunches of venison over his shoulder, the other gobbling breakfasts of partridge pie, cold mutton, truffles, and a dozen plover's eggs and kedgeree, washed down with a pint of claret.

While not having such a regal appetite, I assumed that my problem was greed. But my assumption was contradicted when I began to measure the energy equivalent of fat on which all diet books based their calculations. Diet books start from the position that the energy equivalent of a pound of fat is 3500 calories (or, to use the exact term, "kcal").

Thus, Audrey Eyton, in *The F-Plan Diet*, instancing a woman whose normal energy requirement is 2000 calories a day:

> If we were to put you on a slimming diet providing you with 1500 calories a day, you would be 500 calories short of your requirement and these would have to be taken from your body fat. It has been scientifically estimated that a pound of your own body fat provides approximately 3500 calories. So during a week you would be likely to shed one pound of surplus fat.

And, by the same calculation, anyone who not only abandons the F-Plan but also consumes 500 calories too many will gain one pound of surplus fat every week.

John Durnin, Professor of Physiology at the University of Glasgow, has told me that this calculation is inaccurate. It is based on laboratory experiments made a hundred years ago that do not take account of the biochemistry within the human body. He says that

> losing one pound of fat would result in a net energy deficit nearer 3000 kcal. More important, because the mechanical and biochemical efficiency of depositing adipose (fatty) tissue is relatively inefficient, you need about 4500 kcal to lay down one pound of fat in the body.

A TANGERINE TOO MANY?

Even allowing for Professor Durnin's correction (a reminder that human chemistry is more subtle than the chemistry conducted in laboratories on inert material), many of us would indeed be gross. An extra 4500 calories a week is just under 650 calories a day. According to Dr. Fox's BHMD, 650 calories may be composed of:

Hamburger, broiled, regular, 3 oz.	245
Potato chips, 2 inch diameter, 10 chips	115
Beer, 12 fl. oz. (2)	300

Or, from a standard textbook:

Chocolate, plain (3.5 oz.)	525
Peanuts, salted (25 gm)	150

Or, from Audrey Eyton's "F-Plan Calorie and Fiber Chart":

Cake, fruit, plain, average slice (2)	400
Oatmeal cookie (4)	280

So, according to these figures, a couple of snacks a day over the limit in a café or bar or at home will result in the consumption of food with an energy content of 650 calories or more.

In this case, if the diet books are to be believed, anyone who eats this quantity of food in addition to daily requirements will gain one pound of fat a week, which is to say over 50 pounds a year, or over 500 every ten years.

I seemed to gain about 12 pounds a year. It was difficult to be precise, since when not on a diet I was usually making up weight lost from the previous diet.

The weekly equivalent of 12 pounds a year is about 4 ounces. Assuming these 4 ounces are fat, the calorie equivalent—allowing for Professor Durnin's correction of the textbook figures—is 1125 a week, or 160 a day over my requirement.

So, if my problem was, indeed, that I was eating 160 calories a day too many, the answer should be simple. According to the diet books, I should be able to maintain a steady weight by every day saying "no" to any of the following, give or take the odd calorie:

Cookie, 1 oz. (2)	160–170	(*Which?*)
Yogurt, low-fat, hazel-nut, 5.3 oz.	160	(Eyton)
Martini	150	(Stillman)
Gingerbread, $2 \times 2 \times 2$ in. (1)	180	(Tarnower)
Wine, dessert (4-oz. glass)	160	(Fox)

It is difficult to wrap the brain around the notion that one glass of wine (or a pint of beer) over the limit is evidence of greed. Furthermore, a weight gain of 12 pounds a year is

120 pounds a decade, an increase that would take me from an initial post-diet weight of 160 pounds, say, to 280 pounds. That, of course, was what I feared, the fate to which I believed I was doomed, unless I dieted. British weighing machines often stop at 250 pounds. The thought of going off the scale was a waking nightmare.

The fact is, though, that people who gain fat do not do so at anything like the rate of 120 pounds a decade. A more typical rate of increase, for the man or woman who in time becomes fat, would not be 120 pounds a decade but perhaps 30 pounds. This would change the slim young woman aged twenty weighing 112 pounds into a woman aged twenty-five weighing 127 pounds and into one of thirty weighing 142 pounds who will be worrying about her weight. Likewise, a man who between the ages of twenty and thirty increased from 154 to 184 pounds would metamorphose from being slim to being decidedly overweight and liable to worry about becoming obese in the next decade. (These figures assume sedentary women and men of average height; taller people might gain rather more weight proportionally from a heavier initial weight.)

The energy equivalent of a gain of 30 pounds of fat in a decade is 40 calories of energy from food a day. Forty calories a day? As the diet books count them:

Potato chips, 2-in. diameter (4)	46	(Fox)
Tangerine, raw, 2½-in. diameter	40	(Tarnower)
Butter, 1 pat	50	(Stillman)
Pickle, sweet, 1 oz. (1 rounded tbsp)	40	(Eyton)
Tomatoes, fried, 2 oz.	40–50	(*Which?*)

Most diet books recommend calorie control. Theirs is a world where the dieter is invited to measure potato chips with a ruler and to believe that eating four more than the body's requirements will lead to a weight gain of 30 pounds in a decade (to be exact, close to 35 pounds according to Dr. Fox's calculations, assuming that the chips are round and not elliptical). And eating three less than the requirement—a difference of seven chips—will lead to a weight loss of 30 pounds in a decade.

No diet book has ever made such a claim, because it is

absurd. But there it is: the arithmetic, supposedly based on science, proposes that one tangerine too many, every day, is the path to obesity.

THREE CHIPS TOO FEW?

Consider the arithmetic for the person who eats three chips too few each day. (This amounts to a 2-ounce package of chips once a week.) The consequent and apparently inexorable weight loss would mean that the slim young woman of 112 pounds aged twenty would weigh 22 pounds aged fifty. If she underdid it not by three but by four chips a day, by the age of fifty she would have disappeared altogether.

Consider a different case: the person who does eat or drink quite a lot too much. Take, say, the man who puts away 3 pints of beer and a couple of packages of peanuts a day, on top of eating and drinking enough for his body's needs. (If that is greed, there is a lot of it about.) This extra intake, with a pint of beer at 175 calories and peanuts at 300 calories for 2 ounces, is 1125 calories a day. At the rate of "4500 calories equals one pound of fat" this moderate drinker would gain about 8 pounds a month, or just under 100 pounds every year.

In my dieting days, I never did the sums necessary to show that the reasoning of the diet books advocating calorie control was preposterous. Although calorie counting did strike me as obsessive to the point of being deranged, I took the books on trust. After all, every diet I went on worked. They succeeded. I failed.

I was also concerned about my health. The diet books have ways of keeping the dieter obedient. Dr. Stillman has a chapter entitled "Facts to Help 'Scare' the Fat off You." He quotes Brillat-Savarin: "Well, go ahead and eat and grow fat," the French gourmet said. "Become ugly, heavy, have asthmatic attacks and die choked by your own fat." Or, according to Stillman, Tarnower, and indeed *Which? Way to Slim*, you may well develop diabetes, gallstones, arthritis, strokes, heart disease. "If you're 10 percent overweight," says Stillman, "you'll lose seven years of living. In effect you will have committed suicide at sixty-three." I did not want to suffer or die prematurely. And it seemed the only means of prevention was to eat less.

FAT PEOPLE EAT LESS

John Garrow is often cited as the leading English authority on obesity. He wrote in 1974 that there is "no evidence of any relationship between energy intake and body weight in man." In 1977 at a congress on obesity he said that no evidence had been found "that obese people ate more than thin ones. The cause of obesity is astonishingly difficult to pin down." In 1983 I asked Dr. Garrow if any evidence had emerged since 1977 to show that fat people ate more than thin people. He said no.

In 1974, Professor Durnin, in a study made in Glasgow, found that fat girls did not eat more than thin girls: they ate less than thin girls. Durnin also made two studies of fourteen-year-old boys and girls, in 1964 and 1971. During the seven years, calorie intake had fallen by 180–250 calories a day. In 1971 the boys who were eating less were fatter than the 1964 boys. (Girls stayed much the same.) A more recent study by Durnin, in 1982, showed that what he found for children is also true of babies. Generally speaking, weight for weight, fat babies eat less than thin babies. Nutritionist Alison Paul and others undertook a variation of these studies in 1982 and discovered that today's teenagers eat fewer calories than their parents and, indeed, eat 300–500 calories a day less than is recommended by the World Health Organization. But nevertheless they tend to be overweight.

In 1979, Professor Harry Keen reported on the links between what and how much people eat and diabetes. As part of his study he measured the amount of food people ate, and their degree of fatness, in three population samples: 961 employees of Beechams Foods; 1005 employees of the Greater London Council; and 1488 middle-aged civil servants. What he found, to his surprise, was "highly significant inverse correlations between food energy intake and adiposity [degree of fatness], a relation found in both sexes and in all three population samples."

In other words, the fatter people were eating less than

the thinner people. This applied to both men and women and to all the groups studied. Keen eliminated people who were dieting from his analysis; this did not affect his results. He considered the possibility that the fatter people were under-estimating how much they were eating; but such self-decep-tion is only likely among people worried about being fat, and Keen's study was of people who did not see themselves as having a weight problem. Also, Keen's discovery that thinner people ate more and that fatter people ate less applied right across the range of thinness and fatness, not just to those people who were most overweight. As was to be expected, Keen found that people got fatter as they got older; but the rule that fatter people ate less and thinner people ate more applied to all ages.

In March 1984, I attended a conference of the American Heart Association in Tampa, Florida. Dr. George Sopko of the St. Louis Medical Center reported a "strong inverse relationship between caloric intake and body fatness." His finding was identical with that of Keen: the fatter the people in the study, the less they ate. (Moreover, the thinner people, who ate more, were less likely to die from heart attacks.)

The Royal College of Physicians of London, comment-ing in its 1983 report on surveys of obesity done in the last fifty years, states: "There now seems little doubt that there is a general trend for both men and women to become heavier and presumably fatter, this change being particularly evident in young adults."

As long ago as 1960, the United States Society of Actu-aries, analyzing the statistics of twenty-six large life insur-ance companies, found the frequency of overweight and obesity to be as follows:

Age	Overweight (%)	Obese (%)	Overweight or obese (%)
MEN			
20–29	19	12	31
30–39	28	25	53
40–49	28	32	60
50–59	29	34	63
60–69	28	29	57

Age	Overweight (%)	Obese (%)	Overweight or obese (%)
WOMEN			
20–29	11	12	23
30–39	16	25	41
40–49	19	40	59
50–59	21	46	67
60–69	23	45	68

But while the estimated amount of body fat has continued to rise steadily in the last twenty years, the *National Food Survey,* a British official publication, shows that the amount of food energy consumed has steadily dropped. In 1960 the British people were consuming 2628 calories a day from food in the home. In 1981 the figure had dropped to 2210: a fall of 19 percent. The figures for recent years are:

1960	1965	1970	1975	1979	1980	1981
2628	2590	2560	2290	2250	2230	2210

These figures exaggerate the drop in energy intake from food because they do not reflect the fact that there are now more old people, who tend to eat less, than there were in 1960. They also do not take into account food eaten outside the home, which has increased since 1970. However, the Ministry of Agriculture does publish statistics which include food eaten outside the home. They show that consumption of sugars continues steady, and that alcohol consumption is continuing to rise; but that overall, between 1960 and 1981, there was a drop of over 200 calories per head per day in food consumed.

In the United States, Dr. Theodore van Itallie, a leading American researcher, estimates that since the beginning of this century, the average American eats 10 percent less but weighs 14 percent more.

Whatever the exact figure may be, it is safe to say that we are getting fatter while eating less. Professor Peter Wood of Stanford University, referring to findings from the United States, Britain and other Western countries, confirms that "generally speaking fatter people eat less than thinner people."

But if overeating is not the cause of obesity, so that the very word "obese" (derived from *ob,* "over," and *edere,* "to eat") is based on a misconception, what makes people fat? If not gluttony, then what? The answer seemed to lie in a word not much mentioned in the diet books but which has crept into many women's magazine features lately: "metabolism." The Obesity Research Foundation says:

> The ability of some people to eat what they like and not gain weight is the constant envy of the obese. It would seem that the lean and the obese are metabolically different, and the explanation of the difference is an urgent challenge to science.

My grandmother used to say that fat people had something wrong with their glands; I thought this was a homely way of saying, as is often said now, that fat people have "a low metabolism" or, more correctly, "a low metabolic rate." Was this my doom? Had the great double-dealer in the sky given me an unwinnable hand? Should fat people not be scorned as greedy, but pitied as helpless?

EATING LIKE A BIRD AND LIKE A HORSE

The notion that fat people are burdened with a low metabolism has been popularized by Dr. Robert C. Atkins, whose *Diet Revolution, Super-Energy Diet* and *Nutrition Breakthrough* have sold a total of 12 million copies, worldwide. Dr. Atkins is as enthusiastic about his books as Dr. Stillman and Dr. Tarnower were about theirs. He maintains:

> Failure to lose weight on a diet low in both calories and carbohydrates is strong evidence of a metabolic imbalance. . . . variations in metabolic responses are important factors in obesity, and any physician should know that he will be seeing many cases of impaired response.

Metabolism can be defined as "the sum total of all the chemical reactions that go on in living cells." Metabolic rate is the speed at which the body uses energy, which it needs for the constant process of replacing and renewing cells in all its parts while asleep and at rest; for the digestion of food; and for activity. Most people use most energy not for activity but for the workings of their vital organs—the brain, heart, liver and kidneys especially. Put simply, metabolic rate is the speed at which our bodies work.

It is commonplace, nowadays, for people to describe themselves as having either (luckily) a "high metabolism" or (unluckily) a "low metabolism." The assumption is that we are stuck with the metabolic rate we are born with. The fault is not in ourselves—in our sloth, or greed, or both—but in our genes.

One analogy for metabolism is engine capacity. Thus, a middle-aged woman may have a moped capacity and so eat "like a bird" and yet be plump; whereas a young man with a Cadillac capacity can "eat like a horse" and yet stay lean. And just as mopeds do not turn into Cadillacs, nor birds into horses, the inference is that metabolic rate is inborn.

Interestingly, this determinist proposition is similar to the now discredited theory that we are stuck with the intelligence (IQ) with which we are born. It takes away a sense of personal responsibility for our physical shape and blames the Almighty, or heredity. In my case, my father is fat, whereas his father was lean; so I half-believed that when the chromosomal dice were cast I got the low metabolic numbers. I was a slow burner; I was one of those who gained weight as soon as I "looked at a bun," because I had a low metabolism. My friends and colleagues who ate heartily but evidently gained no weight had a high metabolism.

Another analogy often used for human metabolism is the central heating system. Hence the concept of the "appestat." Yudkin says: "You could more or less describe the appestat as the part of the brain that controls how much we eat in the same way that a thermostat controls temperature." But "if you are overweight, you don't stop wanting to eat when you've had enough. So obviously something has gone wrong with your appestat."

The thermostat that controls the temperature of my

bathwater is set at 135° F., just as the thermostatic mechanism that controls the temperature of my body is set at 98.4° F. But if the thermostat of my water heater was stuck at 145° F., it would be too high and would have gone wrong.

With this analogy in mind, a number of scientists, aware that fat people do not characteristically eat more than thin people, have proposed the "set-point" theory. This supposes that people who tend to obesity suffer from a condition in which the mechanism that regulates their body weight is set too high. As a result they tend to gain weight.

A champion of set-point theory is Professor Richard Keesey of the University of Wisconsin. Keesey works with rats. He says:

> Laboratory animals, like human beings, appear to regulate body weight around a stable level or set point. If their weight is reduced by restricting their calorie intake, rats rapidly restore body weight to the level of nonrestricted controls when allowed to feed freely. . . . Thus, as in man, the stability and vigorous defense of its body weight by the rat suggest the presence of a set-point regulator.

The implication of this ingenious theory is that my weight was never meant to fluctuate; that it might go down when I dieted but would always go up again; and that if I left well enough alone and ate what I wanted, my weight would stop at some point, and stay steady at that "set" point. If I'm fat, it's because I was born to be fat.

BORN TO BE FAT?

In *The Dieter's Dilemma,* Dr. William Bennett and Joel Gurin have popularized set-point theory. They say:

> Some individuals come with a high setting, others with a low one. Some are therefore naturally fat and others thin. Going on a diet is an attempt to overpower the body's set point; it is not a fair contest. The set point is a tireless opponent.

"Your setting," they go on, "is the weight you normally maintain, give or take a few points, when you are not thinking about it.

"The set-point theory is, admittedly, somewhat fatalistic," say Bennett and Gurin. But it does have charm. It suggests that the dieter's real problem is the refusal to accept that she or he is designed by nature to be fat. Love it! "The obsessive drive to be thin serves no real purpose, except to funnel large amounts of money into the diet industry," they say. And: "The prejudice against fatness is cruel, destructive, and unfair." They find support from the "Fat Is Beautiful" movement in the United States and also from Susie Orbach, whose book *Fat Is a Feminist Issue* quite rightly sees tyranny in the pressure put on women to become super-slim.

Was there, then, truth in what my grandmother told me? Was I born to be fat?

Set-point theory does not, however, explain why the average body-fat content of the adult population has increased by 10 percent in the last forty years. And, in any case, is it true that "most of us remain at essentially the same body weight," as set-point theory proposes?

No, it isn't. Set-point theory was discredited before many people had heard of it, let alone believed it. In 1974 a survey of long-stay prisoners in Wormwood Scrubs, whose body weight was measured annually in the eight years between 1965 and 1972, was published in *Obesity and Energy Balance in Man,* a book by Dr. John Garrow, who explained:

> It may be that long-stay prisoners are not typical of the general population, but on general grounds one might expect that their weight would be more stable than that of the population at liberty; their way of life is more like that of laboratory animals which show great stability of body weight.

And the results of the routine weighing of these prisoners? "On average their weight varied over a range of 7½ kg (16½ pounds) during a period of seven years."

Garrow supported his findings by quoting studies of more than 1000 people in Wales which showed weight deviations over four years of more than 20 pounds; and of the community of Framingham, Massachusetts, in which "on average, both men and women fluctuated by 10 kg (22 pounds) over eighteen years."

So much for set-point theory. Man is not a rat.

In 1976, my last year of dieting, I was not aware of set-point theory, but I was no closer than its champions have ever been to finding out why I got fat. If the reason wasn't sloth, and wasn't greed, and wasn't genes, what could it be?

In his *Super-Energy Diet,* Dr. Atkins calls a chapter "If You Are Not Getting Results." Addressed to hopeless cases, it includes a tip which sounds like the most loony but harmless remedy ever proposed. "A surefire trick if you can afford it," he says, is to "go to Europe." How could this help me? I live in Europe. But Dr. Atkins perseveres:

> For some strange reason, as yet unexplained, a trip to Europe always seems to help with weight reduction. It may be something in the soil. . . . The best results seem to be achieved in Mediterranean countries: Spain, Greece, Italy, or the south of France.

In summer 1979 I had not read Dr. Atkins, and I had abandoned dieting, having decided that I'd rather get fat than go mad. I went to Greece for a vacation and spent a month on Antiparos, a tiny island in the Cyclades. When I left England, I weighed a flabby 180 pounds. When I returned I was down 8 pounds. I later lost a bit more weight, while eating and drinking whatever I wanted. For the first time in my life my weight became stable.

What had happened in Greece? Its clean air had given me a good appetite, but this book does not propose that eating makes you thin.

EXERCISE: THE KEY?

Nor was I taking more exercise than usual in Greece. The reverse was true—for the previous autumn I had started to jog. I had been in Hyde Park, watching the first *Sunday Times* National Fun Run, now an annual event with 30,000 participants. The exaltation of the runners, some almost twice my age, was an inspiration—not to start running to lose weight, but to join in for the fun of it. Watching the runners, and reflecting on an imminent fortieth birthday, I came to three conclusions: I was a spectator of, not a participant in, my own life; there are no easy ways out, and nothing worthwhile is easy; and if I didn't start then, I never would.

So I started to jog. By the next summer I was doing gentle four-and-a-half-mile runs and sometimes covered twenty miles in a week. Then came the Greek holiday, during which I enjoyed walking, and some swimming, and a sense of well-being earned by my new fitness that I'd never experienced before as an adult. But I took no more, and probably less, exercise on that holiday than in the previous months. Afterwards I regarded the weight loss as an enigma.

Since then, running has become part of my life. I still weigh 168 pounds, but I have changed shape. And talking with many people about the effect of exercise on weight and fat, I have found plenty who, like me, started running when 10 to 30 pounds too heavy, lost weight, lost fat, and now eat and drink what they like. It was when I realized that I would never again have to diet that I started the research for this book.

2

Dieting Makes
You Fat

The Holy Grail of Western medicine is a safe and comfortable way to lose excessive body fat. This fruitless search has been the basis of an almost endless array of "reducing diets" that have tantalized the fat folks and enriched the publishers and the medical businessmen. The reducing diets have been disappointing—some would say, a medical disaster.

—George Mann
New England Journal of Medicine

It was not through statements that we learned how to breathe, swallow, see, circulate the blood, digest food, or resist diseases. Yet these things are performed by the most complex and marvelous processes which no amount of booklearning and technical skill can reproduce. But we have been taught to neglect, despise and violate our bodies, and to put all our faith in our brains. As a consequence, we are at war within ourselves—the brain desiring things which the body does not want, and the body desiring things which the brain does not allow; the brain giving directions which the body will not follow, and the body giving impulses which the brain cannot understand.

—Alan Watts
The Wisdom of Insecurity

THE BIG SLOWDOWN

A successful diet book is liable to sell millions of copies worldwide. For many people, their desire to lose weight matters as much as anything else in their lives. They are not doing it for fun, and therefore they are entitled to expect that any writer of a diet book will have at least an elementary knowledge of the effects of dieting on the human body. But do they?

As a rule, diet books are based on two assumptions about dieting. The first is that diets do not affect the speed at which the body works—the metabolic rate. The second is that weight lost on a diet is all or almost all fat. "When you are slimming you are really eating your own body—eating away the part of it you don't want, that surplus fat!" says Audrey Eyton.

It is a pity to single out Mrs. Eyton, because her F-Plan recommends eating foods rich in fiber, which often are nourishing, whereas the foods recommended by other diet books are often disgusting, debilitating or even dangerous. But she is typical of writers of diet books when (having made the "1 pound of body fat equals 3,500 calories" calculation), she says:

> Expected rate of fat loss has always been estimated simply by counting the calories consumed in the form of food, any food, and subtracting them from the number the body requires for energy. . . . With a daily deficit of 1000 calories you could expect to shed around two pounds a week.

Is it true that diets do not affect the speed at which the body works? No, it is not. Diets slow down the metabolic rate. And is it true that weight lost on diets is fat or almost all fat? No, it is not. Much of the weight lost on a diet is not fat; and any initial fast weight loss includes almost no loss of fat.

These facts have been known for many years. Research into the effects of diets on the body started at the beginning of this century, and studies have been repeated again and again. Diet books have so totally ignored this information that it is impossible to believe that all diet books are written in good faith, particularly since the profits to be made from them are so large. Diet books lead their readers to believe that when diets fail it is the dieter who is to blame. But in fact, diets fail because of what they do to the body of the dieter.

What happens to the body depends to a considerable extent on the nature, severity and length of the diet, and also on the dieter's body composition, eating habits and way of life.

First, any diet book that claims or suggests that an initial weight loss of 10 to 15 pounds a week is fat is misleading the reader, as a simple calculation will show. The energy you need to use to burn off a pound of body fat is 3000 calories (Professor Durnin's correct figure). It follows that the energy required to burn off 10 to 15 pounds of fat a week is 30,000 to 45,000 calories, or 4286 to 6429 calories a day. But diet regimes recommend cutting down by only 500 to 1500 calories a day. There is thus no way that the initial fast weight loss, which dieters are led to believe is proof of success, can be body fat. It must be something else.

(Some of the more reckless writers of diet books suggest that the foods recommended on their regimes have a special fat-burning property in addition to their low-calorie value. These claims are nonsense; they have the same sort of relationship to nutrition as astrology does to astronomy.)

RAPID WEIGHT LOSS IS OF GLYCOGEN

The body's first reaction to a diet regime is to draw on the energy that is immediately available in any emergency. This is not fat. The body's immediately available form of energy is a substance that you do not read about in diet books: glycogen. Glycogen is a form of glucose (a carbohydrate) stored in solution with water, in the muscles and in the body's most metabolically active vital organ, the liver.

How much glycogen does the body contain? It is difficult to be exactly sure. Unlike other constituents of the body (bone, or fat, for example) it cannot be dissected, because it disappears after death; and this is a reason why its function has tended to be overlooked until recently.

The Scandinavian physiologists Professor Per-Olof Åstrand and Professor Bengt Saltin have made a special study of glycogen. I asked them, and also Dr. John Garrow, to make an estimate of the body's glycogen content. These three authorities were in broad agreement. First, the body stores glycogen in solution, in the proportion 1:2.7 glycogen to water; second, the amount of "solid" glycogen the body contains is about 2 pounds. It follows from this that the weight of glycogen in solution contained in the body is approximately 7½ pounds.

Glycogen burns very much faster than fat. You have to use up about 3000 (unreplaced) calories to burn off a pound of body fat. In sharp contrast, only about 400 calories are required to burn a pound of glycogen in solution with water. This is because glycogen is a carbohydrate, and carbohydrates burn over twice as fast as fat. In addition, very little energy is required to release water from the body's cells.

So, initial rapid weight loss on a diet is no mystery. The loss consists principally of glycogen bound up with water, as well as additional water. Simple mathematics proves the point. This otherwise inexplicable rapid weight loss is a familiar phenomenon in sport. A footballer playing hard in the sun, or a marathon runner, can lose up to 10 pounds, or even more, in two or three hours. I myself have lost 8 pounds running a half-marathon on a humid day.

A special diet used by marathon runners (the so-called "carbohydrate-bleeding" regime) consists of food specially designed to drain the glycogen stores, and loses about 6 pounds in three days. It is not a calorie-controlled diet; you can eat as much as you like of very high-protein foods such as meat, fish, eggs and cheese. (The runners follow the "bleeding" regime with "carbohydrate-loading" for the three days just prior to a marathon, and saturate their bodies with energy-giving starch.)

The effect is the same as the diet regimens of Dr. Stillman and Dr. Tarnower, which recommend high protein and low carbohydrate; and of Dr. Atkins, which recommends high fat and low carbohydrate. It is these diets which drain the body's own carbohydrate store—glycogen—fastest. The body must have carbohydrate: the brain, for example, uses glucose released into the blood almost exclusively as a fuel and has practically no glucose store of its own.

Low-carbohydrate diets drain the body's glycogen stores in the first few days without touching the body's fat stores at all. British researchers, notably Professor Philip James, recognized this phenomenon first. For in the Royal College of Physicians 1983 report on obesity of which James was chief author, it is stated of diet regimes:

> The patient needs to know that short-term rapid weight losses with rigorous diets depend on losses of body water (with glycogen and protein) rather than on losses of body fat.

Low glycogen levels trigger the mechanism in the body that signals hunger. Foods such as bread, spaghetti, cereals, beans and potatoes are satisfying not just because of their energy content but because they are nutritious, and rich in carbohydrate in whole form, and feed the glycogen stores, raise the blood glucose level, and give a sense of fullness and well-being.

By contrast, a runner on the "carbohydrate-bleeding" regime eats lots of protein and, with a full stomach, loses weight and becomes ravenously, obsessively hungry. This hunger has nothing to do with an empty stomach or a low energy intake, nor is it caused by loss of fat. The cause of the hunger and of the weight loss is exhaustion of the glycogen store, together with water. The surest way to get someone obsessed with food is to put him or her on a low-carbohydrate diet regime.

Glycogen loss leads to low blood sugar levels. The result is a sense of weakness, depression, irritation, tiredness, and sometimes faintness and dizziness. Dieters will recognize the pattern.

At the same time that they lose glycogen bound up with water, dieters also lose water from elsewhere in the body. It is possible to lose 7 pounds of water sweating it out all night in a Turkish bath; I once won a lose-weight contest that way. Boxers and jockeys dehydrate themselves so as to weigh in under a required weight. The human body contains 50 to 65 percent water. Women's bodies contain less water than men's, because body fat contains only a small amount of water, and the average woman has more fat than the average man. For the same reason, a fat person's body contains less water than that of a lean person of the same weight. Water is essential for the body's metabolic processes, but the body responds to a diet by reducing its water content.

FAT PEOPLE STAY FAT

In our minds we know the difference between going on a diet and being subjected to famine or starvation. But our bodies do not know the difference. When we go on a diet we activate the mechanisms in the body that protect us and preserve us in times of famine. And what does the body need to keep it going between times of famine? Fat. The more often people diet, the more their bodies will protect the stores of fat.

The human body can adapt to circumstances. It can get used to very hot or very cold weather, or to high altitude. The body constantly adjusts to accommodate a person's way of life, preserving what that person needs, if necessary at the expense of what is not needed, or at least not used.

Once a dieter's body has adapted to the diet by releasing glycogen and shedding water, it will then tend to lose the tissue it needs least. The body of a sedentary dieter will tend to lose lean tissue, muscle in particular, simply because a sedentary person does not need much muscle. The longer the dieter has been sedentary, the stronger the tendency for lean tissue to be lost. And the body of a fat dieter will seek to preserve fat, simply because it is accustomed to fat. By contrast, the body of an active and relatively lean person, even if it has a great deal of muscle, will tend to lose body fat, simply because the body has been trained to need muscle; it is being used all the time.

There comes a point, even in an almost inert person, at which the body will protect its lean tissue. But this switch takes some time. Physicians can devise diets for anyone which, with persistence, will lose far more fat than lean tissue. But the body's processes include what can be termed "tissue memory." After a crisis, the body will tend to rebuild itself in the form appropriate to the way in which it is used.

Lean, active people who go on a diet—boxers and jockeys, for example—lose weight efficiently, lose fat if they have any to lose, eat a lot after dieting in order to refuel and tend to gain muscle, the body having adapted to their way of life. (Heavyweight boxers who go to fat do so because in training they may be so active that they can eat up to 7000 calories a day. Out of training they often continue to eat a great deal of food without being sufficiently active to consume the energy from it.)

Most dieters are not boxers or jockeys but are fat, inactive people who tend to lose relatively more lean tissue than fat.

ADAPTING TO A DIET

Dieting also slows the body down. First of all, a dieter is likely to become less active without necessarily even noticing. You may sleep a little longer, walk up stairs less often, not feel like tackling an energetic task, find that the television programs have suddenly become very good, or just spend more time sitting and musing. In these situations the dieter is often not aware that a pattern of inactivity is forming, as the body seeks to make do with less food.

On the other hand, a dieter may realize she or he is less active—"I'm taking it easy, I'm on a diet." The result can be a pleasant sense of restfulness or an unpleasant sense of lassitude, but for the body, the results are the same.

Dieters do not normally take to their beds. During any but the most rigorous diet, activity is not usually dramatically reduced. But a man may use 150 to 450 calories a day less if he is more sedentary; a woman maybe 100 to 300 calories less.

Also, the less food you eat, the less energy you need to digest it. A diet that cuts 500 calories a day needs about 50 calories a day less energy for digestion. It follows, therefore, that if fairly active people cut 500 calories a day, their bodies need not lose significant amounts of fat, or of any other body tissue. The body of a fairly active person can adapt to a moderate diet by becoming the body of a sedentary person.

In practice people on a mild diet; if they keep to it, will lose some weight and also some fat. But they cannot lose a pound of fat a week by cutting 500 calories of food a day, or anything like that amount, unless they consciously compensate for the body's adaptation to the diet by becoming more active.

The reason many diet books specify an energy intake of only 1000 calories a day for women and 1500 calories a day for men (or levels of this order) is that the body needs more energy than this for its basic, vital functions.

At rest, it is the vital organs that have the most work to do. The brain accounts for about 20 percent of the body's energy used at rest. The liver is even more active, accounting for about 27 percent of the body's activity at rest. The contribution of various parts of the body to energy turnover are estimated to be as follows:

Liver (and associated areas)	27%
Brain	20%
Heart	7%
Kidneys	10%
Skeletal muscle	18%
Remainder	18%

At rest, then, about 65 percent of the energy the body needs is used by vital organs whose weight totals about 5 percent of the body's weight. Of the remaining 35 percent, some is used by body fat, which, like the rest of the body, requires nourishment and constantly renews itself. Most of the remaining energy is used by muscle, which is more active than body fat. How much more active depends on the condition of the muscle. The little-used muscles of a sedentary person are relatively inactive at rest. Muscle regularly used, say by someone who exercises vigorously three or four times a week, is relatively active at all times, not just during exercise. This is because the stress of exercise breaks down muscle tissue, and the muscle then actively regenerates. During exercise, the energy used by muscle increases dramatically by twenty, fifty or even a hundred times more than the amount used at rest, depending on the condition of the muscles and the intensity of the exercise.

The regularly used muscles of an active person are, with training, able to use more and more energy, and to burn more and more fat.

A sedentary person's body uses most of its energy from food for the vital autonomous functions (which happen unconsciously). In addition, the average healthy able-bodied sedentary person in our society will need maybe a quarter as much again for the processes of conscious living: sitting down, talking, writing; and somewhat more energetic activities, such as standing, walking around the house and the office; household chores; and holidays spent mostly on the beach. This, of course, is an outline of a typical Western lifestyle.

As already mentioned, the process of digestion itself uses about 10 percent of the energy from food. So, for example, 2500 calories eaten a day require about 250 calories for digestion; 1500 calories eaten a day require 150 for digestion.

So a fair estimate of the total energy needs of a sedentary person can be produced: 65 percent for the body's autonomous functions, another 10 percent or thereabouts for digestion and roughly 25 percent for all other activities of living. A sedentary man of 154 pounds will be in energy balance (meaning that he will tend to stay the same weight) eating around 2400 calories a day. The equivalent figure for a woman of 120 pounds is around 1700 calories a day. The figures, in round terms, are:

	Rest (calories)	Digestion (calories)	Living (calories)	Total (calories)
MAN (154 pounds)	1700	250	450	2400
WOMAN (120 pounds)	1200	200	300	1700

These figures are substantially below those recommended by the World Health Organization for people defined as "fairly active": people who take some trouble to compensate for having sedentary jobs, or people, such as postmen, whose jobs involve walking around a lot, or those who engage in regular active recreation like gardening, tennis or golf. For such people the WHO figures are around 3000 calories a day for the 154-pound man under fifty years old, and around 2200 calories a day for the equivalent 120-pound woman. But even these "fairly active" people use a lot more energy when asleep and at rest than when active.

DIETING SLOWS YOU DOWN

On a diet, the body of a fairly active person can thus accommodate a drop of a few hundred calories by becoming much less active. But the body of a sedentary person does not have so much room for maneuver. And in any case, diet regimes usually provide only 1000 to 1500 calories a day or less.

How does the body accommodate such a sharp cut? The diet-book theory, which might seem common sense, is that the body has no option but to lose fat. But as already stated, the body has many other options. Not only can it lose glycogen, water and lean tissue and slow down its waking activity, but its vital functions can slow down as well. The dieter's metabolic rate, like that of anyone who fasts or who is starving, slows down to adapt to the new situation.

The diet books have ignored the scientific studies of this phenomenon, although it is well known to specialists in obesity and energy balance. The fact that human metabolism is not static but dynamic, and that it is depressed by dieting, is such vital knowledge that it is worth describing in some detail the studies that have proved the point.

THE SCIENTIFIC EVIDENCE

People who believe that dieting works have often said to me, "But nobody ever got fat in a concentration camp." This macabre fact is presented in support of the idea that the voluntary semistarvation of dieting will reduce overweight people to some point short of emaciation. Images of skeletal people on hunger strike, or of the victims of famine, also seem to serve as evidence that dieting works.

Dr. Marian Apfelbaum, of the Bichat Hospital in Paris,

investigated what happened to the people of the Warsaw Ghetto during the two years of famine in the Second World War. It is known that their average daily calorie intake was between 700 and 800: maybe 1700 calories a day less than they consumed before the famine.

It is safe to assume that the average weight of body fat (also known as "adipose tissue") in an adult is about 30 pounds, representing roughly 100,000 calories. A deficit of 1700 calories a day for two years amounts to a total deficit of 1,000,000 calories, in round figures: "approximately ten times the equivalent in energy of the adipose stores," as Apfelbaum says. What, then, happened to the remaining deficit of 900,000 calories?

A less extreme but better-documented case is of 700 Swiss whose calorie intake was measured between 1942 and 1946. In 1942 the average intake was 2400 calories a day, as it was in 1946. In the intervening years, food restrictions forced the intake down to 2100 calories a day, then 2000, then 1850. The accumulated deficit was 600,000 calories per person. But the average weight loss for the whole period was 20 pounds a person, which, measured as body fat, amounts to 60,000 calories. What happened to the remaining 540,000 calories?

Apfelbaum reviewed these cases of forced restriction of food because he was concerned with:

> The problem of an obese person who loses weight on a restricted diet but then stops. Physicians in the past have tended to say that such a patient must be a liar, because they considered that energy expenditure was not influenced by energy intake. I think they were wrong.

And he concluded: "There is a wealth of evidence showing that there is a reduction in energy expenditure with restricted diet." That is to say, dieting slows down the metabolic rate.

The classic experiments on the physiology of dieting were carried out in the United States by F. G. Benedict in 1919 and by Ancel Keys in 1945. Benedict put thirty-four student volunteers on a diet, first of 2100, then of 1500 calories a day: as healthy young men their normal requirement was 3100 calories. The goal of the experiment was to achieve a weight loss of 10 percent, which took sixty days. But their metabolic rate declined to a greater extent than this loss of body weight could account for: by 18 percent.

Keys' project was more ambitious. He restricted thirty-six volunteers to a diet of 1570 calories a day for a longer period: twenty-four weeks. The volunteers were highly motivated, as they were conscientious objectors who felt it appropriate to deprive themselves. At the end of twenty-four weeks their weight had on average declined by 24 percent. But their metabolic rate at rest had declined by 39 percent. Like many women dieters, these young men also damaged their health.

The outward signs of this loss of vitality were lethargy and apathy. The young men lost interest in themselves, in each other, in sex and in visitors. They stopped spontaneous play and avoided work. Two had mental breakdowns. All became obsessed with food.

Some studies, including one recently made by Dr. John Garrow and co-workers, of nineteen very obese women who lost an average of 66 pounds in a year by means of jaw-wiring, have shown a drop in resting metabolic rate matched by weight loss. But grossly obese people, who may suffer from inborn errors of metabolism, or whose bodies may be wrecked by constant dieting, are unreliable subjects. The studies of people on restricted diets in less extreme circumstances, corresponding to the situation of all but the most obese dieters, consistently support the findings of Benedict and Keys: the drop in metabolic rate exceeds the drop in weight.

George Bray, Professor of Medicine at UCLA, put six overweight women on a diet of 450 calories for twenty-four days. He reported in the leading medical journal *The Lancet* that their weight dropped by an average of 22 pounds, a drop of 7 percent. But their energy expenditure dropped by 15 percent.

Dr. Apfelbaum recently reviewed the results obtained in twenty-four studies of undernutrition made between 1903 and 1969. Men and women of widely varying weight and in different circumstances were underfed for different reasons for periods varying between three weeks and two years. "All the authors report a decrease of the basal metabolic rate ranging from 10 to 45 percent according to the length and stringency of the [diet] restriction."

Derek Miller of Queen Elizabeth College, London, Audrey Eyton's nutritional adviser, strongly criticizes the theory that, as he puts it, obesity is caused by "either or both of the deadly sins, gluttony and sloth." He is convinced that "energy intake and expenditure influence each other."

Like Apfelbaum, Miller contradicts the notion that dieters who say that they eat little are lying. He took thirty veteran dieters from slimming clubs to Ragdale Hall, an isolated country house. Their luggage was searched and their car keys taken away, and they were fed a diet supplying the same number of calories as Benedict and Keys gave their young male volunteers: 1500 a day. Miller's regime lasted for three weeks. The metabolic rate of these seasoned dieters was so low that "although nineteen subjects lost weight, nine maintained within plus or minus a kilogram (2.2 pounds) and two actually gained weight."

Derek Miller believes that he is now hot on the trail of what, for some, might prove the richest prize in obesity research: a patentable drug to speed up the metabolic rate. It is worth remembering that the two most common methods currently used to speed up the metabolic rate are smoking and amphetamines—both addictive, and more damaging to health than obesity. Doctors I have spoken to believe that there is no such thing as a safe drug that speeds up the metabolic rate.

Meanwhile, a famous statement made by Professor Albert Stunkard, a leading researcher at the University of Pennsylvania, still holds good:

> Most obese people do not enter treatment for obesity. Of those who do enter, most will not remain. Of those who remain, most will not lose much weight. Of those who lose weight, most will regain it.

THE DANGERS OF DIETING

How does the body slow its metabolic rate? The dramatic drop in metabolic rate produced by the experiments described could not be caused by loss of fat, because fat is a relatively inactive part of the body. Obviously it is more efficient to slow the function of the body's most metabolically active cells: those in the vital organs. Ancel Keys proposes just such a mechanism, and it might well give any dieter pause for thought:

> It appears that the tissue loss and the changes in the metabolic rate of the liver and other organs with high metabolic rate may be of considerable importance in explaining the changes in basal metabolism during starvation and food restriction.

And he calculates that 80 percent of the decrease in oxygen consumption in his subjects can be accounted for by a halving of the oxygen used by the liver and its associated organs.

The body needs oxygen all the time for its vital functions. The greater the body's capacity for oxygen, the fitter a person will be. A high capacity for oxygen protects against diseases of the heart, lungs and blood vessels. But the consequence of dieting, Keys proposes, is to lower the body's use of oxygen dramatically. Thus, dieting can hardly be a healthy activity.

Professor Stunkard confirms that dieting slows down the metabolic rate and frustrates the dieter. He goes on to say: "Repeated attempts at weight reduction may lead to a progressive slowing of weight loss and to even more rapid regaining of weight."

I have yet to read an account of this phenomenon in any diet book. This is not surprising. The facts that the scientists have known for decades, and that have been set down in scientific journals and textbooks, make most diet books so much waste paper.

Now, the medical establishment is beginning to acknowledge that metabolism is dynamic. The Royal College of

Physicians, referring to some of the studies summarized here, put a bomb under the diet books by saying, in their report on obesity:

> It has been known for many years that there are substantial differences in the metabolic rates of individuals at rest and also that the body is able to adapt to changes in energy intake. If volunteers are given only half their usual intake, there is an early fall in the metabolic rate of the tissues.

And in April 1984 *The Lancet* summarized: "The normal response to a diminished food intake is a disproportionate decrease in resting metabolic rate." Dieting slows you down more than weight loss can explain because dieting slows down the processes of the most active vital organs in the body. This process can be dangerous if the diet is extreme or prolonged or unbalanced, or if the dieter is not in good health, or if the dieting is repeated over a number of years. Millions of people, women mostly, go in for fad diets every year. They are damaging their health.

The more severe the diet, the more you slow down. Fasting has the most dramatic effect. "Energy requirements decrease by 25 to 30 percent in the course of three to four weeks of fasting," reports Ernst Drenick, an American doctor who favors fasting as a treatment for obese patients. He goes on to say:

> Restraint should be advised in the amounts of food allowed after fasting or after the desired weight level has been attained with fasting. The adaptive lowering of the metabolic rate may quickly lead to substantial weight gains if normal, average meals are consumed during this period.

In other words, the only way not to put on the weight that has been lost by fasting is to go on a diet after the fast has ended.

FASTING WASTES MUSCLE

Drenick subjected 137 very fat people to fasts of between one and four months. The average weight loss was 64 pounds. The patients were well pleased. However, when 105 were followed up two years later, ninety-six had regained their pre-fast weight. Drenick acknowledges that during two-month fasts his subjects lost 17 pounds of muscle on average, but he does not suggest that this is why they regained weight. Instead, he says that "regular revisits and close supervision" during the follow-up period are crucial and concludes:

> Our experiences are disappointing. [But] a sizable number of the subjects had been on welfare for years; many of them had never been usefully employed. Therefore solid motivation over the long run might be questioned in some of these patients.

In other words, the experiment is valid, but the subjects are not up to standard—a new version of "the operation was successful, but the patient died."

Sometimes, fasting results in death from heart failure. So does fasting modified by the administration of liquid protein, a regime made popular in America by Robert Linn's book *The Last Chance Diet*. In 1978 the American government investigated fifty-eight cases in which this liquid protein diet had led to death from heart failure. The more extreme a diet is, the more dangerous it is.

But what happens to patients who do survive fasts? Frederick Benoit, a California doctor, subjected seven fat U.S. naval personnel to a fast short enough to tempt impatient dieters: ten days. In this time the average weight lost was just over 20 pounds. However, of the weight lost, two-thirds was lean tissue and only one-third was body fat. Benoit concludes that "fasting beyond ten days may produce decreasing rates of lean tissue breakdown" but "the wisdom of incurring such wastes in lean body tissue is open to question."

There is something to be said for fasting. People who occasionally fast for a day or two often find the experience refreshing. But fasting is not a way to lose fat. It slows down the body's activity dramatically, to a point as close as ordinary people ever get to hibernation, and it wastes lean body tissue, including muscle, designed to be metabolically active. Fasting changes the composition of the body, so that after the fast the body works at a lower energy level than before it started, not only because weight has been lost but also because of the loss of metabolically active tissue. Special exercises, like those used by physiotherapists to rehabilitate people whose muscles have been wasted as a result of inactivity after a surgical operation, are the only way to restore the body to its previous metabolic rate after it has undergone a prolonged fast.

OVEREATING SPEEDS YOU UP

If dieting slows you down, and fasting slows you down even more, does it follow that overfeeding will speed up the metabolic rate? Yes, it does. Overfeeding does not make you thin, of course, but it does speed up the rate at which the body uses energy. The studies on this subject are as extensive as those on underfeeding.

In 1901, a German, R. O. Neumann, reported the results of an experiment upon himself, in which he overate for long periods. After an initial weight gain, he found that he could eat 800 calories a day above his normal intake and gain little extra weight. His conclusion was that "someone who is healthy can take in surplus food and consume it by burning it faster."

This experiment was repeated by Derek Miller in the 1960s, when forty-nine subjects were encouraged to eat at least 1000 calories a day above their normal intake for periods of up to eight weeks.

> There was a marked weekly adaptation to the calorie load, such that the rate of weight gain fell throughout the experiment.

After overfeeding, a person's metabolic rate when asleep and at rest speeds up, as does the energy used as a direct result of eating. Most remarkable of all is the effect of overeating on the energy used when exercising. Oxygen consumed during exercise is a measure of energy used. In one study the oxygen consumed by people who were overeating increased by 30 percent during walking, 25 percent during cycling and 19 percent during stair-climbing. By contrast, Ernst Drenick found that after a three- to seven-week fast, oxygen consumption decreased by 21 percent during bed rest, 32 percent when sitting, and 40 when walking. The human body will always adapt to circumstances, and seek balance.

Diets train the body to adapt to the circumstances of dieting, which it does by slowing down its vital functions. This adaptive behavior is the best means of staying alive and as healthy as possible in famine. Our minds know the difference between going on a diet and famine or starvation; but our bodies do not.

DIFFERENT PEOPLE, DIFFERENT SPEEDS

Different people have different metabolic rates, for a variety of factors that help to explain why some people never get fat and other people get fat very easily. These include physical makeup, mental state, the circumstances in which people live, and their state of health; how active they are; and how fit they are. Not only is metabolism dynamic, slowing down or speeding up according to the volume of food eaten; it is also variable by choice. Dieters feel imprisoned in their bodies partly because they do not realize that they can speed up their metabolic rate. Within wide limits we can choose how much energy we want our bodies to use; it is literally a question of how lively we choose to be.

Other things being equal, a heavy person needs more energy than a light person. Someone who loses weight will use less energy and need less food simply because of being lighter. A tall person needs more energy than a short person because a larger body surface enables more heat to escape.

Because body fat is metabolically less active than fat-free tissue—muscle and vital organs in particular—the greater the proportion of fat-free tissue in the body, the more the energy requirement. Similarly, the greater the proportion of fat in the body, the less energy is required. This means that other things being equal, a lean person needs more energy from food, and uses more oxygen, than does a fat person.

Men are not only usually heavier and taller than women, but also usually have less body fat. The average woman has around 9 percent more body fat than the average man. There are three types of body fat: subcutaneous, deposited under the skin; depot, lying deeper, characteristically on the belly in men and around the hips and thighs in women; and essential fat, within the body to protect the vital organs. Women have more depot and essential body fat than men. The average man uses more energy than the average woman not because he is a man but because he is heavier, taller and leaner. A woman and man of the same height, weight and body composition will have much the same energy requirements.

ENERGY BREEDS ENERGY

From adulthood onward, energy requirements decline by about 4 percent a decade. It follows that the average sixty-year-old requires about 20 percent less food than the average twenty-year-old. The World Health Organization's recommended figures for daily energy intake from food are:

Age	Men, 154 lbs. (calories)	Women, 120 lbs. (calories)
16–19	3600	2400
20–29	3200	2300
30–39	3100	2200
40–49	3000	2200
50–59	2800	2000
60–69	2500	1800
70 +	2200	1600

It is true that maximum oxygen capacity, a measure of physical energy requirement, declines slowly as a function of age, at a rate of about 2 percent a decade. But these figures mostly reflect the fact that the amount of exercise people in the West do take declines almost to zero in middle age. People who remain active into old age continue to need, and to use, high amounts of energy. Elderly Swiss farmers of both sexes have been observed to have an energy requirement as high as 4000 to 5000 calories a day.

As a rule, adolescents require more energy than adults, for their growth as well as their activity. Pregnant women need about 300 extra calories a day; and lactating women about 500 extra calories a day.

The sedentary man or woman who becomes less active but eats more in middle age is in trouble. Having recognized that the role of physical activity in weight gain in middle age has up to now been underemphasized, the Royal College of Physicians report on obesity states:

> Increasing inactivity in middle age forms the basis
> for the decline in muscle mass and lean body mass
> as people grow older.

To say that people have a high metabolic rate is to say, in scientific terms, that they use a lot of energy. An energetic person uses those parts of the body that are metabolically active and will therefore need and use more energy at rest and when active. Diet books discourage us from taking account of what, given reflection and self-awareness, we already know: energy breeds energy.

LOW ENERGY AND DEPRESSION

Mental and emotional states, and physical health, also affect the speed at which our bodies work. Being "high" or "low" is not just a mental state; it reflects high or low biochemical states. Elation and fever are two examples of high states, one good, one bad; both require and use more energy. Depression literally depresses the body's energy. People in low mental states may gain fat not because they eat more food, but because the food they are eating, normally the right amount, is too much for a depressed state. Depressed people who worry about weight but are unaware that depression affects the rate at which the body uses energy are caught in a vicious circle. Lacking guidance, they are liable to eat a normal amount of food, gain fat, and so become more depressed. If a pattern is established, the result may be self-destructive behavior, such as eating abnormally large quantities of food ("bingeing").

People in industrialized societies have lost touch with their bodies. When animals are out of sorts or physically depressed, for whatever reason, they spend a lot of time resting and sleeping. So do people in tribal societies. The body has its own energy resources. Pressing food on someone who is ill is usually the wrong thing to do; the body's energy needs to be directed to the source of the illness, not to digestion.

The common experience of one particularly strong emotion, the state of "being in love," is that the lover refuses food when he or she is secretly pining after the loved one. If Romeo and Juliet wanted to lose weight in the first part of their play, they were in luck. But when love has the lineaments of gratified desire and is altogether active, not passive, then the Tom Jones syndrome applies, and the lover is liable to eat with the appetite of the furnace in a steam locomotive.

To recognize the physical, mental and emotional circumstances that determine and change metabolic rate really requires nothing more than common sense.

LEAN PEOPLE USE MOST ENERGY

The more you weigh and the more lean body tissue you have, the higher your metabolic rate will tend to be at all times—when asleep, when resting and when active.

The tables of energy requirements from food, such as those published by the World Health Organization and in books of nutrition, give body weight, together with age, as the only factors affecting resting metabolic rate (that is, the speed at which the body works at complete rest, just after sleep). In one crucial respect these tables are misleading. They imply that heavy people have a high metabolic rate and so require more food simply because they are heavy; and that light people have a low metabolic rate and so require less food simply because they are light. This is actually only half the story.

What dieters especially should know is that the people who have the lowest metabolic rate are people who, as well as being light, are also fat; and that the people who have the highest metabolic rate are people who, as well as being heavy, are also lean. Of course, it is true that, more often than not, light people are lean and heavy people are fat. But this is not always the case. A tall male manual worker may be a muscular, lean 196 pounds. A middle-aged sedentary woman may be no more than 112 pounds, but if she is no more than average height, she may be very flabby; that is to say, she may have little lean tissue and much fat on her body.

It follows that a light, lean person can have the same energy requirement as a heavy, fat person. Professor John Durnin has calculated that it is possible for a lean person weighing 112 pounds to need and use the same amount of energy as a fat person weighing 154 pounds. The table below is recalculated from Professor Durnin's book *Energy, Work and Leisure,* and shows, in round figures, the amount of resting energy needed per day by people not only of different weights, but also of different body compositions.

Resting Metabolic Rates, in Calories

MEN	WOMEN	112 lbs.	133 lbs.	154 lbs.	175 lbs.	196 lbs.
Lean		1450	1650	1850	2050	2250
Average	Lean	1300	1500	1700	1900	2100
Fat	Average	1150	1350	1550	1750	1950
Obese	Fat	1000	1200	1400	1600	1800
	Obese	850	1050	1250	1450	1650

In this table, an "average" man is equivalent to a "lean" woman because, as stated, women have more body fat than men. Thus, a lean man has around 10 percent total body fat; a lean woman, around 20 percent. Likewise, a "fat" man, as here defined, has about 30 percent body fat; a "fat" woman, about 40 percent.

FAT PEOPLE USE LEAST ENERGY

What these figures show is that (to take extreme cases) a fat person of 112 pounds (the shortish middle-aged woman) has a resting requirement of 1000 calories of food a day; a lean person of 196 pounds (the tall manual worker) requires 2250 calories of food a day. Now, assume that the woman is sedentary, but not unusually so, and uses 25 percent above her resting metabolic rate for activity. Also assume that the man uses 1800 calories of energy a day because of his work (which is roughly accurate if he is working fairly vigorously for six hours a day). The figures, in round terms, come out as follows:

	Rest (calories)	Digestion (calories)	Living (calories)	Total (calories)
Lean man (196 pounds)	2250	450	1800	4500
Fat woman (112 pounds)	1000	150	250	1400

Thanks to Professor Durnin's calculations, it is now clear why an active man can, indeed, "eat like a horse" and yet stay lean, while an inactive woman can, indeed, "eat like a bird" and yet gain weight and fat. The figures show why Derek Miller's experiment had the result that it did; for some women 1500 calories a day can take them over the top.

What these figures also show is that a big, active person can take more liberties with food than can a small, inactive person. The fat 112-pound woman will be eating more than twice her daily exercise requirement if she eats a couple of slices of cake, or four cookies over the limit. Indeed, the same applies to a young woman who drinks an extra orange juice and also an extra soft drink in one day. By contrast the lean 196-pound man can have six extra 12-ounce cans of beer and yet be consuming only half as much again as he normally requires. All he needs to do to get back in energy balance is to lay off the french fries for a couple of days, or else go for a run.

The people who are most unfortunate of all are women who have put themselves through diet after diet throughout their adult lives. As a result they will slowly but surely have wasted their metabolically active lean tissue; they will have lost the ability to take exercise; and they will, quite likely, be artificially light yet artificially fat, because of the futile misery they have put themselves through. Such women could literally be obese weighing only 130 pounds, and gain fat eating no more than 1500 calories a day. It is impossible for such a woman to be healthy, for reasons explained in the next chapter ("Sugar Makes You Hungry").

An inactive woman of 112 pounds cannot transform herself into an active man of 196 pounds. But suppose a fat, inactive woman of 112 pounds became a lean, active woman of 112 pounds, choosing a new life which involved an extra 750 calories of energy a day in exercise. How would the sums look then?

	Rest (calories)	Digestion (calories)	Living (calories)	Total (calories)
Fat woman (112 pounds)	1000	150	250	1400
Lean woman (112 pounds)	1300	250	1000	2550

Weight for weight, a lean woman can eat more than 1000 calories a day more than a fat woman. The taller and heavier the woman, the greater the contrast. And here is the answer to the diet books. Active people can eat the equivalent of a meal a day more than inactive people, and stay lean, while the inactive people continue to get fat.

FAT REGAINED

If a fat woman of, say, 154 pounds could, by dieting, reduce to 112 pounds, and if the diet worked according to her dream, so that all the weight lost was fat, then she could eat almost as much food at the lean weight of 112 pounds as she previously did at the fat weight of 154 pounds. But this dream is a fantasy which—as most dieters know—is liable to become a waking nightmare.

As a rule, any diet that has resulted in a loss of 10 or 15 pounds in the first week or two will result in a gain of the same amount a few months after the diet has ended. A crash diet lasting a few days that results in a loss of, say, 6 pounds will result in that weight being regained as fast as it was lost, if not faster.

It is of course true that any diet prolonged over a period of weeks will result in a loss of fat, together with glycogen and water, and metabolically active lean tissue. But the loss of nonfat tissue has the effect of lowering the body's energy requirements.

If a dieter is prepared to follow a prolonged diet with what is in effect a modified diet for life, then, indeed, it is possible to keep lost weight off. Millions of women do just that. The cost is depression, weakness, exhaustion and permanent malnutrition caused by deprivation of the food a body needs to be healthy. However, if people become a lot more active after a diet, then they can not only keep lost fat off, but also eat more and grow leaner. The reasons are fully explained in a later chapter ("More Air! More Air!"). The only people I know who in the long term have kept much weight off after a diet has ended are those who started to exercise regularly during or after the diet.

However, most people regain the weight lost on a diet. Weight Watchers and *Slimming* magazine (founded and then published by Audrey Eyton of *The F-Plan Diet*) promote newspaper and magazine features and publish books graphically showing massive weight loss of dieters who have used their methods. Commercial slimming clubs are not, however, noted for long-term follow-up studies. Nor, it must be said, are doctors. In 1979, Rena Wing and Robert Jeffery of the University of Pittsburgh Medical School completed a review of 145 dieting projects involving 6927 patients, published between 1967 and 1977 with medical supervision. Of these, only eight included a follow-up one year or more after the project was "complete." Indeed, only forty-three included a follow-up of any duration at all. The reason, of course, is that diets do not work, and that people responsible for the administration of diet regimes do not want to admit to themselves, and certainly not to the overweight people who come to them, that the treatment will almost certainly fail. Like casinos, slimming clubs advertise their rare winners.

Very few people indeed eat sparingly immediately after a diet has ended. Almost invariably they respond to the body's cravings by eating at least as much as they ate before the diet started. This is not because of habit, nor, however much the dieters may blame themselves, because of greed, stupidity or thoughtlessness. The body needs energy to regenerate, and responds to the first days after a diet has ended with signals of extreme hunger.

And woe to the sedentary dieter. Once the glycogen and water has been replaced, the body of the sedentary person, being used to fat, will tend to regain fat and will rebuild less muscle. The proportion of lean tissue in the body decreases; the proportion of fatty tissue increases. This is one of the reasons why dieting makes you fat.

Nobody ever became fat in a concentration camp. But the survivors of concentration camps who resumed sedentary lives did tend to get fat. Prison-camp diets devastate muscle. The people who survived Hitler's death camps frequently became very flabby after the war—not necessarily heavy, but fat.

The consequences of a single diet regime, even if severe and prolonged, need not be damaging. The change in composition of the body after one diet is unlikely to be dramatic. All the same, Dr. Garrow's comment on Benedict's sixty-day and Keys' twenty-four-week experiments is a warning to any optimist willing to trust to willpower:

> It is interesting that the volunteers for the semi-starvation experiments of Benedict et al. (1919) and Keys et al. (1950) tended to over-eat and become obese after the termination of the experiment.

In both cases "semi-starvation" consisted of regimes of 1500 calories a day. After his experiment was over, Keys put his subjects on a gradual refeeding program, of the kind all diet books recommend as sensible. The men remained ravenous. After the refeeding program ended and the men could eat as much as they liked, some became ill from overeating; they averaged a consumption of 5000 calories a day, and they regained their pre-diet weights without regaining all their muscle tissue. They began slim, they ended obese.

ENERGY LOST

For the sedentary person a lifetime spent on and between diets is not only self-defeating but also dangerous. Every diet trains the body to slow itself down, losing some lean tissue and not replacing all of it. Cumulatively the composition of the body alters drastically.

Another reason why dieting makes you fat is that fat is lighter than muscle. The net result of a diet, for a sedentary person, may be a loss of weight. But the body of such a dieter may nevertheless contain a greater proportion of fat. Certainly any sedentary dieter who regains the weight lost after a diet is bound to be fatter than when the diet started, simply because she or he will have replaced heavier muscle with lighter and bulkier fat.

A third reason why dieting makes you fat is that fat is less metabolically active than muscle. The greater the proportion of fat in the body, the lower the metabolic rate of that body and, therefore, the less energy required from food.

For a sedentary person, the one sure way to slow the body down and so create the conditions for getting fat is to go on a diet. Every diet trains the body to become less energetic, to require less energy from food, and to use less oxygen. Habitual dieters are on a downward spiral which remorselessly reduces their vitality.

This is why dieting makes you fat.

But why does as much as half the population of the United States, Britain and other industrialized societies steadily gain weight and fat throughout life? Why do we get fat in the first place?

3

Sugar Makes You Hungry

The aspects of things that are most important for us are hidden because of their simplicity and familiarity. One is unable to notice something—because it is always before one's eyes. We fail to be struck by what, once seen, is most striking and most powerful.

—Ludwig Wittgenstein
Philosophical Investigations

Breathing at my side, that heavy animal,
That heavy bear that sleeps with me,
Howls in his sleep for a world of sugar,
A sweetness intimate as the water's clasp.

—Delmore Schwartz
"The Heavy Bear That Goes with Me"

WHY DO WE GET FAT?

Nobody wants to be fat. Most people over the age of thirty acknowledge that they'd like to lose some weight. That is why diet books have such massive sales.

People in industrialized societies have tended to get fatter and fatter during this century. Every year scores of millions of people go on diets, which don't work. Scores of millions more get fat without going on diets. A year never goes by without a representative body of scientists or doctors in the United States or Great Britain stating, again, that obesity is a massive public health problem. An American team of experts with a sense of humor recently worked out that the U.S. adult population was carrying a total of 2,297,000,000 pounds of excess fat, which, if converted into energy, would be enough to supply the annual residential electricity demands of Boston, Chicago, San Francisco and Washington.

It was not always so. Dieting is almost entirely a twentieth-century phenomenon. One hundred years ago and more, few people dieted—because they didn't need to. Few, other than the rich (whose faces are commemorated in paintings) and dandies like Byron, tended to get fat. And dieting is almost entirely confined to the Western world. There still are many millions of people living away from Western influence—hunter-gatherers, pastoralists, farmers, peasants, and people in remote countries—who may eat well, and live to a ripe old age, but do not tend to gain weight as they get older. In the Third World it is usually only when people move from the countryside to the towns, or when they start to eat Western-influenced food, that they put on fat. In these countries, it is the rich (whose pictures we see in the papers and on television) who most commonly get fat.

Diet books and most obesity textbooks assume that we get fat because we are eating more and more. Some people, of course, do get fat because they eat great quantities of food. But greed is not the usual reason. Overall, people in the West are eating less and less while becoming fatter and fatter. What, then, can be the cause of our overweight?

The massive difference between the food we eat now and the food eaten by almost everyone before this century is primarily one of quality, not quantity. Measured in the conventional way, we eat about the same proportion of protein as do people in the Third World who live in settled societies; rather less carbohydrate; and a great deal more fat. The most impressive difference, though, is between whole food and processed food. In particular, all studies made of the differences between the foods eaten in Western and non-Western societies show that people in the West eat great amounts of processed carbohydrate, sugar especially; whereas people who live away from Western influence, including people in Western countries which are little influenced by industrialization, eat great amounts of whole carbohydrates, starch especially.

It makes sense to inquire whether the connection between processed carbohydrates and fatness is causal or merely coincidental.

THE RISE OF THE SWEET TOOTH

Until recently sugar was a luxury. In A.D. 1300 a pound of sugar cost a year's pay; it was then a chic item on the tables of the cosmopolitan rich, much as cocaine is today. In 1700, Great Britain was importing 20 million pounds of sugar a year; in 1800, 160 million pounds. Sugar was, of course, the main nonhuman commodity of the slave trade, and helped to make Great Britain the richest and most powerful nation in the world. By 1850, consumption of sugar had risen to about 20 pounds a person a year. The tax on sugar helped to pay for the Crimean War. In 1874, Gladstone removed the tax on sugar, and consumption rose steeply, so that in 1900 every man, woman and child in Great Britain was eating an average of 72 pounds of processed sugar a year, and expenditure on sugar matched that on bread. The British sweet tooth was bred a century ago. Other countries followed.

Consumption of sugar has continued to rise during this century, except during the two world wars. By the mid-1950s, with sweets no longer rationed, the British were eating more sugar than ever before. According to John Beckett of the British Sugar Corporation, who is in a position to know, the sales of processed sugars "have been almost absolutely stable" for the last thirty years. The figure for Britain in 1955, cited by Mr. Beckett at a conference of the world sugar industry in 1979, was 2,850,000 tons; in 1970, 2,875,000 tons; in 1978, 2,850,000 tons. This amounts to somewhat over 100 pounds a year for every man, woman and child in Britain. In the United States the figure is quite a lot higher; Mr. J. W. Tatem of the American Sugar Association, at the same conference, said that the total U.S. consumption of processed sugars was 128 pounds a person a year.

The average consumption of processed sugars in Great Britain and the United States is therefore between 2 and 2½ pounds a week, a head. On average, sedentary people obtain around 20 percent of their energy in the form of processed sugars.

Many people confuse "sugars" with "sucrose." Nowadays, processed sugars include sucrose, maltose, glucose (notably in Britain), fructose, and high fructose corn syrup (notably in the United States). Watch out for these names on food labels. From the health point of view they all amount to the same thing, as do all versions of brown sugar. The industry calls the stuff "refined." Here it is correctly called "processed."

The world average consumption of processed sugar of all types is now about one-third of the Western figure. The overall African figure is about one-fifth, but is rising. The overall Asian figure is about one-eighth, but is also rising. Wherever Coca-Cola and Pepsi-Cola signs can be found, more and more sugar is being eaten.

There was a time when the British ate more sugar than any other nation; that time has long passed. People in Mediterranean countries still eat less of it; but people in North America confront sugar-saturated food at every meal.

In America, three-quarters of all sugar eaten is contained within manufactured food, and of this well over half is in chocolate, candy, cakes, cookies and soft drinks. Chocolate is over half sugar; sweets are almost all sugar. Cookies vary between 10 and 45 percent sugar; soft drinks such as Coca-Cola are about 90 percent water and 10 percent sugar (meaning that all their calories are sugar).

Some Americans eat less, some more, than the average of 128 pounds a year of sugar. Adolescents who snack a lot and young men and women without the means or inclination to prepare their own meals may eat 200 pounds a year, or even more, which means that close to half the energy they get from food can come from processed sugar.

To someone without a sweet tooth the figure of 128 pounds a year of processed, "refined" sugar may seem remarkably high. But sugar is used extensively by food manufacturers in foods not generally thought of as sweet, as one of the lists at the end of this chapter (page 100) shows. Sweet pickle is about one-third sugar. Canned fruits with syrup total about one-quarter sugar, as does tomato ketchup. Many ready-to-eat breakfast cereals are even heavier in sugar. Flavored and fruit yogurt is between 13 and 18 percent sugar; baked beans can be anywhere from 5 to 15 percent sugar. Varying amounts of sugar are added to soups; diluted with an equal amount of water, condensed cream of tomato soup is over 5 percent sugar. Anyone who wants to avoid eating processed sugar has to be alert.

There is now a trend toward eating less sugar at home, but more away from home. In Great Britain, Mars Bars, the most popular candy bar, were first manufactured in 1932. Fifty years later, 700 million were sold. Between 1932 and 1982 the amount of candy eaten per head went up from 5½ ounces to 8 ounces a week—the extra 2½ ounces is the weight of one Mars Bar, which contains 320 calories.

While naturally occurring sugars in fruits and in some vegetables are nutritious, processed sugar has no nourishment in it. It is inert. It contains no vitamins and only the faintest traces of some other nutrients. Of all the foods we consume in any quantity, it is comparable in this only with alcoholic spirits. It supplies dead, or empty, energy. And the very last food that is suitable for a basically sedentary population is food that supplies nothing but energy. Almost all brown sugar also contains no nourishment. Only in sugar accurately labeled "raw cane" sugar does some nourishment remain.

We have been taught that the principal requirement of the human body is quantity: readily measurable energy. This is wrong. Our principal requirement is quality: nourishment, which is not so easy to measure.

The advertisements for products sweetened by sugar foster the notion that the energy in food is used mostly for activity. This is not true. As stated in the last chapter, the lightly active person, who compensates for a sedentary job by walking, gardening, golf or any other regular weekend and holiday activity, uses only one-third of energy intake for activity; the other two-thirds go to fuel the body's basic functions, and digestion. And our bodies need nourishment from vitamins, minerals and other nutrients, not merely energy.

Throughout this century, people in Western countries have become less active. The automobile and the elevator have replaced walking. Machines do housework and gardening. Much work on the farm, in factories and on building sites has been automated. People even buy electric carving knives. And yet, at the same time, more and more of the food we eat has nourishment processed out of it, and, in the case of processed sugar, contains no nourishment at all.

LOW ENERGY, POOR NOURISHMENT

I asked Arvid Wretlind about the consequences of this. Professor Wretlind, a world authority on vitamins, works for the National Institute of Public Health in Stockholm and has made a special study of the nutrition problems of people who consume small amounts of food.

He pointed out that men and women still need the same levels of vitamins and minerals as they did before the twentieth century. Until this century, people obtained nourishment from food supplying 2500 to 3000 calories a day or more, because their regular physical activity required a calorie intake at that level. Wretlind explains:

> The lower the physical activity the higher will be the content of the essential nutrients required per calorie in order to obtain the desired, optimal, nutritional level. A diet which is adequate for a man with a calorie requirement of 3000 calories a day cannot simply be assumed to cover the desirable nutritional supply for a low calorie consumer—for example, a woman with a calorie requirement of less than 2000 calories a day.

That is to say, people with low energy intake need to eat especially nutritious food to have any chance of getting enough vitamins and minerals. Studies show that varying groups of people with a low energy intake receive insufficient nutrients, for example vitamin A (carotene), riboflavin (vitamin B_2), vitamin C (ascorbic acid), calcium and iron. Wretlind's conclusion is:

> The low caloric group, such as schoolgirls, office girls, women, and old-age pensioners, do not receive a supply of nutrients corresponding to that considered desirable for good nutritional conditions.

Here he is describing healthy people of normal habits, or, at least, superficially healthy people, for he goes on to say that in Western countries, "a number of disturbances occur in the state of health and well-being which are either wholly or partially due to the unsuitable composition of the diet or to defective dietary habits."

When you think about it, the implications are apparent. Take an average-size woman who, before this century, would have been in energy balance eating nourishing food with an energy value of, say, 2500 calories. The equivalent woman of the same height now, who has an office job, will be in energy balance at about 2000 calories a day, even if she takes a little exercise. Therefore, she can only be getting 80 percent of the nourishment her body needs.

Now assume she is eating an average amount of processed sugars, supplying, say, 400 calories daily. It follows that she cannot be consuming more than 1600 nourishing calories daily. She is therefore getting at most only two-thirds of the nourishment her body needs. I would call that a state of mild chronic malnutrition, suffered not only by sedentary women but by men with office jobs, too.

Processed sugars are not, though, the only food we eat that is short of nourishment. The process of milling white flour from whole grains results in white bread that is robbed of most of the vitamins and minerals naturally present in wheat. The same applies to white rice and to any pasta that is not whole wheat. Much "brown" bread is not much more than colored white bread. (Good bread is "whole wheat" or "whole meal.")

Even worse, we in Western countries eat an average of 40 to 42 percent of our calories in the form of fat, compared with the 30 percent that was the average around the turn of the century. The body needs fat, but far, far less than the amount we eat. Peasant communities in the Third World do well enough eating around 12 percent of their calories as fat. Not only do we eat far too much fat, but we also eat a lot of animal and other saturated fats in the form of convenience food which, like white bread, is drained of nourishment. In moderation, for example, butter fresh from the farm is a healthy food. Butter "blended" with additives, and then stored in a butter mountain for longer than the consumer can imagine, is not healthy food. Refrigerated, fats remain eatable—just—for a long time. But in that time much of what nourishment remains after the process of manufacture disappears.

Viewed as a business commodity, the ideal food is cheap, is easily transported, does not rot, preserves other foods and is highly palatable. Food is processed not in order to be more nourishing but in order to become a better commodity—to make more money. All manufactured foods lose nourishment. And food advertised as having vitamins and minerals added is usually food which has lost more vitamins and minerals in the process of manufacture than are later added back.

WE GET FAT IN ORDER TO STAY HEALTHY

Yet more nutrients are lost in the process of preparation and cooking. Generally speaking, the more sophisticated these processes, the more nourishment is lost. (The original meaning of "sophistication" was "adulteration." Brewers in previous centuries who "sophisticated" their beer with sugar were fined or beaten.) Japanese food, celebrated as among the most healthy in the world, is undercooked. We in the West discard much of the most nutritious parts of food—skin, peel, pith from fruit and vegetables, blood and guts from meat. Then we overcook what we choose to eat, with the result that the water-soluble vitamins B and C go down the drain and many other nutrients go up in smoke.

At the same time that the food we eat is depleted of vitamins and minerals, the environment of the twentieth century has, if anything, increased our need for them. The body uses vitamins partly as a means to ensure a healthy immune system—to resist disease. The more poisonous our environment is, the more vulnerable we are to infections and other noninfectious diseases. These days our earth, our air, and our food are all contaminated. We cannot tell exactly what effect defoliants sprayed on the soil, carbon monoxide from cigarettes and from exhaust fumes, and hormones injected into the animals we eat have on our health. We can, though, be sure that these toxic substances, together with the drugs we take and the thousands of chemicals that are legally added to foods, are draining our bodies of vitamins.

None of this takes dieting into account. What happens when people who are normally getting only about half the nourishment their bodies need go on a diet supplying, say, 1000 calories a day? Unless the diet eliminates all sugars, saturated fats and other highly processed food, in favor of fresh, lightly cooked and nourishing food, their bodies will suffer a sharp shock and will be jerked from a state of mild malnutrition into acute, even severe malnutrition.

From the body's point of view, the significant change is not the drop in energy intake; we have always been able to adjust to scarcity and famine, by means which frustrate the dieter. The starvation that the weight-conscious dieter suffers is not of energy but of nourishment.

Here is another reason for the raging appetite dieters develop after the diet has ended. (This compulsion for food can so baffle and overwhelm dieters that it becomes a genuinely frightening experience.) The healthy body can adjust to a period of emergency, which in effect is what a diet is; but, once the emergency is over, the body's imperative demand is for the nourishment that succors it.

Without being greedy, we are liable to consume more energy from food than our bodies require, because this is the only way our bodies can get enough nourishment. We become overweight against our will, as a means of staying healthy. Overweight people who are always in a good mood are people who have come to terms with being fat. Their well-being springs not from weight, but from the fact that they get enough nourishment from food. Such people tend to level out at a weight and percentage of fat well above the "desirable" level, but they do get adequate nourishment.

When sedentary or even moderately active people eat sugars and other highly processed foods the only way they can get enough nourishment is to consume more energy than their bodies require. A vigorously active person can burn off these extra, empty calories, a less active person cannot. Sedentary people will eventually become overweight and then fat; or they can choose to be undernourished, in which case they will suffer from malaise, and ultimately illness. Ironically, though, becoming fat is, in time, also likely to bring illness with it.

"Sugar is an unnecessary source of energy in a community with such a widespread problem of overweight," stated the Royal College of Physicians in its 1983 report on obesity. The report *Dietary Goals for the United States,* published in 1977 (best known as the McGovern report), came to much the same conclusion. The Royal College report went on to confirm that sugar is not only without value but also deprives us of the vitamins and minerals we would eat in healthy food displaced by sugar:

> A halving of the average sugar consumption per head of the population would increase the nutrient/energy density of the diet. This would ensure that mineral and vitamin requirements were more likely to be met.

Why a halving? Members of the Royal College working party have confirmed to me that their report recommended a halving of processed sugar consumption, rather than cutting it out altogether, for practical, not medical, reasons. The Royal College sees its responsibility as including not only the public and the doctors, but also the government, which does not welcome reports hostile to the interests of the food industry. There is a limit beyond which no representative body is likely to go, in making radical proposals. The same problem exists in the United States: the Reagan administration has sought to block many of the McGovern proposals. Nevertheless, independent and medical experts' reports in America, many European countries and Australia have made it clear that we have no need of processed sugar and that it deprives us of vitamins and minerals we do need.

DEFICIENCY STATES

What are the consequences of eating processed sugar? Deficiency diseases are caused by lack of nutrients; by malnutrition, usually, not merely undernutrition. In the past, some diseases caused by lack of vitamins became epidemic among groups whose food was very unbalanced, often because of unnatural living conditions, as among the newly industrialized poor, or on board ships.

Scurvy (caused by lack of vitamin C, also known as ascorbic acid) was commonplace among British sailors, often causing more deaths than battle or shipwreck, until lemons and limes were found to prevent it (hence "Limeys," the American slang term for the British). Scurvy remained fairly common among poor people who ate no vegetables in wintertime; and rickets (caused by lack of vitamin D) was a common disease among the children of the urban poor until fifty years ago. Xerophthalmia, caused by lack of vitamin A, or carotene, results in blindness in many children in the Third World, especially Africa. Beriberi, caused by lack of thiamine, or vitamin B_1, still occurs, particularly among people in Asia whose staple cereal is processed white rice. Pellagra, caused by lack of niacin (nicotinic acid, or vitamin B_3), was rampant in the southern states of the United States among people whose staple food was corn.

These are the "classic" deficiency diseases, caused by lack of vitamins we have long known about. More vitamins are being identified all the time. The B vitamins, which include riboflavin (B_2), pyridoxine (B_6), folic acid (also known as folate), cobalamin (B_{12}), and pantothenic acid, tend to work with each other while also having particular vital purposes. Lack of them causes corresponding deficiency states and diseases, which have been found particularly among people who eat mostly processed food.

In their clinical form, caused by gross malnutrition, deficiency diseases are easy to diagnose. But deficiency states also take mild forms that are not readily identifiable. Dr. Donald McLaren, in his standard textbook *Nutrition and Its Disorders,* says:

> Malnutrition means disordered nutrition. Nutrition becomes disordered as a result of any deviation from normal. While gross deviations give rise to frank clinical signs and symptoms and definite biochemical abnormalities it is virtually impossible to draw a line between "normal" and "abnormal."

In common with a growing number of doctors and scientists who have made a special study of the subject, McLaren states that large numbers of people in Western countries are short of vitamins and minerals. Surveys have shown, for example, that 36 percent of American women and 26 percent of Swiss women are short of pyridoxine (vitamin B_6). One reason for this is that the contraceptive pill leaches B_6 from the body. One cause of spina bifida is almost certainly lack of folic acid, B_6, B_{12} and zinc supplied to the baby in the womb in the first weeks of pregnancy.

Deficiency of folic acid and zinc is particularly common in Western countries. A nutritionist at the University of Surrey told me that 60 percent of a group of people she examined were short of folic acid, and 30 to 40 percent were short of B_6. And she was studying young athletes who ate a lot of food—much of it, though, junk food. American surveys have shown that around a quarter of the population is short of zinc, calcium and magnesium.

What does "being short of" a vitamin or mineral mean? Panels of doctors and scientists assembled at the request of governments all over the world have made recommendations about the amount of vitamins and minerals people need. These are usually known as RDAs ("recommended dietary amounts"). RDAs are determined by calculating the amount needed to avoid manifest clinical deficiency disease, and adding an arbitrary extra amount "for safety." For example, in Britain the RDA for vitamin C is 30 mg a day, on an estimate of 10 mg a day to prevent scurvy, and 20 mg more to be on the safe side. In the United States the RDA for vitamin

C is 60 mg a day; in the U.S.S.R. it is 75 mg a day. The British government has not got around to asking doctors and scientists to recommend RDAs for most vitamins and minerals. The record in the United States is better, but far from perfect. Of all Western countries, the British are uniquely backward in grasping the connection between food and health.

Surveys commissioned by the British Department of Health state that all but very small subsections of the British population are well fed and get enough vitamins and minerals with their food. Other surveys, however, continue to show that a very large percentage of the British population are short of vitamins or minerals.

Professor Michael Crawford, who is responsible for the welfare of the animals at the London Zoo, has pointed out to me that in most cases the recommended dietary amounts of vitamins and minerals specified for farm animals is, weight for weight, higher—sometimes much higher—than for people. The same is true at the zoo. It is literally the case that what the government says will do for people is reckoned to be inadequate for dogs, pigs, or apes. I asked Professor Crawford for an explanation. "At the zoo," he said, "we are concerned with optimum nutrition." And farmers cannot afford to husband unhealthy animals.

THE NEW MALNUTRITION

Physicians acknowledge that a high percentage of their patients complain of unspecific ailments. These include stomach discomfort, loss of appetite, anxiety, backache, constant tiredness, muscle weakness, jumpiness, digestive trouble, headaches, inability to sleep, difficulty in paying attention, nervousness—or "general malaise," as millions of doctors' certificates put it. Any of these conditions is depressing; all zest for life and sense of well-being is lost. All these complaints can be a result of malnutrition. Most people in Western countries do not eat enough nutritious food, and some large groups of people, including students, office workers, old people and dieters, are especially at risk.

Scurvy is generally assumed to have vanished before the end of the sailing-ship era. Not at all. In its mild form, scurvy leads to bleeding, notably from the gums, and to fragile bones. Later the joints and muscles bleed, and teeth fall out.

Vitamin C is used by the body to resist attacks from poisonous substances, such as lead, cadmium and carbon monoxide from exhaust fumes and from tobacco smoke. Smoking is estimated to lower the vitamin C content of the blood by 25 to 50 percent. Alcohol has a similar effect. So have some drugs—aspirin, for example. The more we are exposed to drugs, poisons and contamination in the air and in our food, the more vitamins we need.

Moreover, foods lose nourishment by being grown in poor soil; by being picked before they are ripe; and by being preserved, dyed or waxed. And no scientist can say what effect the cocktails of chemicals we all eat and breathe are having on our health.

Faced with these facts, confusion and despair tend to set in. What can we do? Short of becoming a crank, an organic farmer or a fugitive from Western culture living on a Greek island, what we can do, today, is to stop eating the one substance that does us no good and can only do us harm: processed sugars.

THINK TWICE ABOUT SUGARS

Sugar causes deficiency states, especially in sedentary people, because it replaces nourishing food, and because it is a parasitical agent, draining nourishment from the body.

Take beriberi and pellagra. Vitamin B_1 and vitamin B_3 are lost in cooking, and are attacked by alcohol. They are also both attacked by sugar. Alcoholics have been diagnosed as suffering from early stages of beriberi and pellagra. Beriberi, or polyneuritis, causes tingling in the hands and feet, mental confusion, and, eventually, heart failure. In mild forms it causes fatigue, weight loss and loss of appetite, exhaustion and sleeplessness, bad memory and mood swings. Mild pellagra, which is in some respects like mild beriberi, has been confused with schizophrenia. Every vitamin has a corresponding deficiency disease; every deficiency disease is likely to have mild forms often not obvious to doctors, and often made worse by drugs.

It may very well be that mild forms of deficiency diseases (also known as "subclinical deficiency diseases" or "deficiency states") are so common in the West that both the sufferers and their doctors fail to see what the problem is. If I feel ill but nobody else does, I know I have a problem. But if a lot of people feel fairly ill all the time, everybody starts to assume that the condition is normal. How often have you heard somebody who is obviously fit, well and happy described—wryly or enviously—as "disgustingly healthy"?

IT'S NOT ALL IN THE MIND

Young people, who consume a great deal of convenience and "junk" food with a high processed sugar content, are especially at risk. Dr. Derrick Lonsdale and Dr. Raymond Shamberger of Cleveland, Ohio, noted among a group of youngsters symptoms of vitamin B_1 deficiency so severe as to be recognizable as an early form of beriberi. Their report emphasized the conclusion that their patients were ill from the effects of eating "empty" or "naked" calories—energy without nourishment.

The doctors noted severe restlessness during sleep, frightening dreams and recurrent fever diagnosed as infections. In a typical case:

> The patient was described as unusually irritable, sensitive to criticism, becoming angered easily and showing poor impulse control, as in the case of a seventeen-year-old male who had put his fist through a plate glass window.

Lonsdale and Shamberger even translated a Japanese treatise on beriberi into English, finding that many aspects of the disease, "forgotten in societies where it is believed that the condition is extinct," imitate other well-recognized diseases, because beriberi affects all the organs and deranges energy metabolism.

How then is it possible to know whether a patient has vitamin B₁ deficiency, rather than some other ailment? The answer is, of course, in the treatment. The youngsters were given vitamin B₁ supplements—and all of them improved.

> Some patients lost their craving for sweet-tasting foods and beverages, although in some cases the process was extremely difficult and the temptation to succumb quite similar to that seen in people who express a wish to stop smoking.

The common assumption that diseases of malnutrition only occur among poor people eating simple food is wrong. Just as beriberi in the East was and is caused by eating white rice, rather than the cheaper brown rice, so Lonsdale and Shamberger's patients were all-American kids eating all-American food.

> Many of them had no breakfast at all; most had school lunch and an evening meal was provided at home. In most cases it was between-meals snacking of so-called junk foods and above all the consumption of a variety of sweet beverages that provided the empty calories.

The consumption of large quantities of soft drinks may well be a danger to health not yet identified in the United States and other Western countries, and it may be that eating and drinking a lot of junk food can cause intensely disturbing changes in personality and behavior which parents, teachers and doctors now label "adolescent."

Hyperactive children can be a great trial to their parents and their teachers. Sometimes such children are diagnosed not only as being disturbed—which, indeed, they are—but also as in need of complex, expensive psychoanalytical treatment. With luck and resourceful parents, a hyperactive child may calm down in time. Others may behave in ways that get them classified as delinquent and then, with the passage of time, as criminal.

In common with such children, most of the people who spend periods of their lives in prison eat bad food. They are likely to have broken homes—and may have come from broken homes. They will find it very difficult to get regular work. They are unlikely to have learned the skills of cooking. It is even likely that the food they eat in prison is more nutritious than the food they choose for themselves. A growing number of doctors and nutritionists, especially in America, are now convinced that certain types of criminal behavior, especially of a bizarre and unpredictable nature, are caused by junk food, and processed sugars in particular. The argument is that the bad food makes these vulnerable people feel bad, and they then act their feelings out.

It sounds unlikely. But, as with the Cleveland study, there is a way to test the theory: give these people good food. Recently in Washington State, California and Virginia, adolescent and adult prisoners were given diets composed of whole food. Their behavior was monitored as, over periods of weeks or months, they were weaned off white flour, coffee, salted foods, and—in particular—sugars. Violence, aggression and other misbehavior decreased, in some cases dramatically. This work has also been done in Britain by the Rev. Vic Ramsey, who, between 1977 and 1980, treated around fifty long-stay drug addicts. Initially with great skepticism, Ramsey and his wife took the patients off convenience foods such as beefburgers, and other foods saturated with salt and sugar, and gave them lightly cooked, fresh whole food. Ramsey said:

> There were colossal changes in behavior patterns when we gave them good food. They were less aggressive verbally, less violent, less refractory.

I asked John McCarthy for his views. McCarthy is ex-governor of Wormwood Scrubs prison in London, and now director of the Richmond Fellowship, designed to help mental welfare and rehabilitation of prisoners. He said:

> If you are under severe stress, one of the best ways to deal with it is to eat healthy foods. I don't need to be convinced of the psychological changes that can

be induced by eating healthy foods. I've seen it all the time.

THE JUNK-FOOD SYNDROME

Growing boys and girls need significantly more energy from foods than do adults, both to fuel their bodies' growth and for exercise, games and sport. Adolescents who are not especially active nonetheless need about 300 calories more than they will five years later. A growing mid-teenage boy who plays a lot of football, say, or other sports will be in energy balance at a level of perhaps 4000 calories a day. A girl of the same age who dances at discos three nights a week will require maybe 3000 calories a day.

Many teenagers who consume a lot of junk food could be in danger of deficiency states. But usually they are comparatively healthy; they eat nutritious food as well, and they do not have enough money to smoke or drink a lot, or consume a great deal of junk food. And there is the pressure of the law and parents' disapproval.

At the age of seventeen or eighteen, all this is liable to change—dramatically. College students and young office workers are at even greater risk from deficiency states. When the body stops growing, and if young people stop taking exercise, they will require perhaps 1000 calories a day less from food. The only way to be sure of staying healthy when changing from a growing active person to an adult sedentary person, sometimes literally from one month to the next, is to eat nothing but nutritious food.

Typically, this is exactly what students and young office workers do not do. No longer obliged to play games, often living away from home for the first time, with parental influence replaced by often rather ramshackle ways of life, in a milieu where far more drinking and smoking goes on, and with little money, young adults turn to the food that is cheapest and most available.

Students, especially, resist eating institutional food, but rarely have adequate cooking facilities of their own. So there is a sharp rise in the consumption of very energy-heavy foods with high sugar and fat content: chocolate, cookies, chips, peanuts with salt, fried food including chips, soft drinks and colas, take-out foods and beer.

A sedentary person cannot burn off the empty energy in these foods, as an active person can. Sedentary adults who eat a lot of sugar are likely to be badly nourished, and diets can put them in a state of acute malnutrition. But the student or young office worker, whose body is unaccustomed to low energy intakes, and who often eats two or even three times the average amount of junk food, is liable to be in an even worse state. If these young people go on diets, they are in danger of acute illness, which may take a mental or physical form.

My son, Ben, when at university, made a habit of cooking fresh food and even of cleaning up after himself. He was regarded with a mixture of awe, puzzlement and derision by the other students and was known by them as "mother." I asked him to list the malaises and ailments of his fellow students. These included what is often known as the students' syndrome: depression, confusion, torpor, inability to concentrate, sleeplessness, mood swings, aches and pains, colds, discomfort in the gut, premenstrual tension, pallor, sweatiness, and an overriding sense that nothing matters. Sophisticates call all this "existential angst." Usually it is caused not by failed love affairs, bad marks or the bomb, but by junk food, and processed sugar in particular.

When I was at university I did not suffer from malaise and ailments. I ate enough nutritive food on top of sugar-heavy foods and gained 35 pounds in three years. I stayed healthy by getting fat. Young women at college or in their first jobs often go the other way. They stay thin while eating more sugar and become ill for lack of nourishment. Ben took another route: he got healthier at university by eating well and being very active physically.

Mothers concerned for the well-being of their children leaving home would do well to ensure that their sons, as well as their daughters, know what good food is and how to cook it. Well-nourished students are far less likely to get depressed.

THE RISE AND RISE OF SWEET FAT

The most popular food sold is saturated with sugar. Nielsen market research shows that the top three food lines sold in 1984 were carbonated beverages, ready-to-eat cereals, and packaged cookies. Also in the top twenty were potato and tortilla chips, ice cream, yogurt, luncheon meats and frankfurters (all of which are loaded with fat, some with sugar).

The energy content of an average-sized potato is about 80 calories; of an apple, about 40 calories. Many of the most popular foods, however, are heavy with calories—not only fats and flour but also chocolate and cookies, chips and sweets. All these are more than five times as high in calories as potatoes, more than ten times as high as apples. Cornflakes almost reach this level; other popular cereals, such as Sugar Frosted Flakes, containing well over half sugar, have a far higher calorie count. Flavored and fruit yogurts, which have something of a "health" image, have a sugar content of 18 percent—rather more than a doughnut.

It sounds sensational to say that millions of people in the West are suffering from mild forms of deficiency diseases, especially when the names of some of the better-known diseases are mentioned—beriberi, pellagra, scurvy. We don't consider malnutrition a problem in the West partly because we associate malnutrition with starvation. But "malnutrition" does not mean "starvation": it means what it says, a state of bad nourishment. And the fact is that most people in the Western world are badly nourished. Moreover, we don't think of dieting as starvation, because starvation is not done on purpose, whereas dieting is. But from the body's point of view there's no difference.

Children, teenagers, students, young office workers, pregnant women and old people are all vulnerable groups of the population, liable to suffer from the effects of eating bad food. For dieters it is even worse, since they are liable, when on the diet, to be in a state of semistarvation.

A rule of thumb for anybody who wants to eat healthy food is: if it's advertised, be careful; if it's canned or packaged, read the label; and if it's got processed sugars in it, don't eat it.

To sum up: eating processed food, and sugar in particular, is liable to make us fat, or suffer the effects of malnutrition. The chronic dieter, yo-yoing from one regime to another, will likely suffer both. That, however, is far from the end of the story.

"WESTERN" DISEASES

The two vital cores of our bodies, central to our health, are the alimentary tract (the stomach and gut) and the cardiovascular system (the heart, lungs and blood vessels). With the first, we process food, and with the second we process oxygen—our two fuels.

In the Third World many people suffer and die from the infectious diseases that have largely been conquered in Western countries by improved sanitation and antibiotics. In Western countries we suffer and die mostly from the so-called "degenerative" diseases of the alimentary tract and the cardiovascular system. Some of these diseases—constipation, piles, varicose veins, obstructions and irritations of the gut, hernias, ulcers, gallstones and diabetes, for example—are inconvenient and can be crippling, but are not usually in themselves fatal. Others—heart disease and cancers—are often deadly. Heart disease is now the biggest killer in the United States, Britain and other Western countries.

In Third World countries not yet touched by Western influence these diseases are rare, sometimes to the point of being practically unknown. They are now known as "Western diseases" or (ironically) the "diseases of civilization" because they spread as Western influence spreads. When Africans come into the towns from the countryside, when Japanese move to Hawaii, when people from the Yemen move to Israel, when Eskimos give up their traditional way of life, when native Americans on reservations accept white life-styles, when people in faraway places have an international airport built in the vicinity, they begin to suffer from the same diseases as Westerners.

Until recently these diseases were generally known as degenerative diseases, because it was believed that they were a consequence of aging, and that people in the Third World were free of them simply because life outside the Western world was short. A similar argument—that Third World people just don't live long enough—has sometimes been mounted to explain why so many people in the West get fat whereas people in the Third World living traditional lives do not.

It is of course true that, in general, life expectancy in Western countries is higher than in the Third World. But life expectancy at the age of forty is much the same in many non-Western countries as it is in the West, and has changed little in the West in the last hundred years. All countries and societies contain plenty of people who live the Biblical three score years and ten, and longer. And the fact is that old people in the Third World, living in the countryside, do not as a rule suffer or die from the so-called "degenerative" diseases. What then is the cause of these diseases, the scourge of Western societies?

FOOD: THE KEY TO HEALTH

Most Western doctors still regard food as incidental to health. But some who have studied the incidence of disease in different societies and countries generally agree that the main cause of the diseases most of us in the West suffer from is the food we eat. One doctor in particular, British Surgeon-Captain T.L. (Peter) Cleave, persistently pursued the connection between Western food and Western disease. During his professional life as a Royal Navy officer, he corresponded voluminously with doctors and scientists all over the world in order to study patterns of disease and nutrition, and he did more than anyone else to bring to public attention the vital role of food in health. If nutrition had its proper, central place in Western medicine, Cleave would have received a Nobel Prize.

In 1956 he published a long paper in the *Journal of the Royal Naval Medical Service:* "The Neglect of Natural Principles in Current Medical Practice." A keen natural historian in the tradition of Darwin, he wrote:

No rabbit ever ate too much grass, no rook ever pulled up too many worms, no herring ever caught too much plankton: no creature in the wild state is ever over-weight. They may vary in size, but never in shape.

He proposed that the key difference between the food we eat and the food animals eat is that much of our food is processed: that is to say, concentrated by machinery and mass-produced.

Wholemeal flour is turned into white flour, and the bran rejected; the pulp of the sugar cane and the sugar beet have the sugar extracted in almost pure form, and the balance of the pulp is then likewise rejected. Now whereas cooking has been going on in the human race for probably 200,000 years . . . there is no question yet of our being adapted to the concentration of carbohydrates by machinery. Such procedures have been in existence for little more than a century for the common man.

Cleave wrote short books on heart disease, stomach ulcers and diabetes in which he traced the rise of these and other Western diseases, showing the link between the diseases and the rise in consumption of Western foods, processed sugar in particular. He also proposed bodily mechanisms by which Western food causes disease. His last book, *The Saccharine Disease,* published in 1974, has had a profound impact on leading doctors in the West. Sir Richard Doll, Emeritus Professor of Medicine at Oxford University, and the man who jointly established the connection between smoking and lung cancer, has repeatedly stated that perhaps 30 percent of all cancers are caused by the food we in the West eat. In a preface to one of Cleave's books Sir Richard wrote that if only a small amount of Cleave's thinking proved to be true he "will have made a bigger contribution to medicine than most university departments or medical research units make in the course of a generation."

Sir Francis Avery Jones, a distinguished doctor who specializes in diseases of the gut, has gone further, saying that the work of Cleave and his supporters "will prove to be, after antibiotics, the most important medical advance of this century."

WESTERN DISEASES ARE NOT "INHERITED"

The title of Cleave's book, *The Saccharine Disease,* reflects his thesis that many Western diseases are properly seen as various manifestations of a single master disease, caused by eating processed, concentrated sugars and starches, which both convert into sugar in the body. Cleave always dismissed the idea, commonly stated by doctors, that Western diseases are "inherited." If so, he points out, why is it that such diseases are virtually confined to people living Western-style lives, and are almost unknown in the wild? Diseases of proven genetic origin are rare; necessarily so, states Cleave, because living creatures evolve in harmony with their environment. Any species in which hereditary defects were common would have become extinct. The fault is not in ourselves, nor in nature, but in our modern man-made lifestyle.

It is true that disease can be transmitted from the mother to the child growing in the womb. Countless animal experiments have shown that the offspring of badly fed females are liable to be born defective or else to develop disease after birth, and to live short lives. In Britain, the official government view is that in general only tiny sections of the population get inadequate nourishment from their food. But in 1982, Professor Michael Crawford and Wendy Doyle of the Nuffield Institute of Human Nutrition in Regent's Park made two studies of pregnant women in London, one in the working-class area of Hackney, the other in the middle-class district of Hampstead. They found that the food of most of the Hackney mothers was short of many vitamins and minerals. As a consequence, their babies were being born light in weight, in some cases so much so as to put them medically at risk for the various physical and mental defects associated with low birth weight. There was no such problem with the Hampstead babies. Much of the food the Hampstead mothers ate was fresh, whereas almost all of the food the Hackney mothers ate was processed sugars and starches together with convenience foods heavy in saturated fats. American studies of deprived inner-city areas produce similar results.

But to say that a disease can be transmitted from mother to child is not to say that its cause is hereditary. Even when a disease is transmitted from generation to generation the cause may nevertheless be something in the environment.

We are all born with constitutions that are more, or less, strong, and with different parts of the body that are more, or less, resilient. People who doubt the causal connection between smoking and lung cancer sometimes refer to the fabulous eighty-year-old man who is hale and hearty on sixty cigarettes a day. If any such man has thrived (and I'm skeptical; he always seems to be someone else's grandfather) he merely proves that some people are born with exceptionally resilient lungs.

Cleave proposed that the environmental cause of various Western diseases is processed and concentrated sugars and starches; above all, processed sugars. Which of these diseases we eventually suffer and die from will largely depend upon our constitutional makeup. Some people will develop stomach ulcers, diverticular disease, cancer of the bowel or other conditions to which they are predisposed by the action of bad food on a sensitive gut. Other people will develop diabetes, heart disease or strokes, because their blood supply has been deranged by bad food. Everybody will develop tooth decay; and very many people will become overweight or obese. Of course, some people will develop clusters of these diseases and disabilities, all of which, Cleave states, are liable to have the same fundamental cause, and all of which rarely occur in people who do not eat the food of the industrialized world.

SUGARS AND THE GUT

Many Western ailments and diseases are harmful to the alimentary tract, or gut. Almost everybody in Western countries is constipated to some extent. It is well known that constipation is caused by a lack of fiber ("bulk" or "roughage") in the food we eat. The condition is eased by eating bran. The basic cause of constipation, though, is that the sugars and starches we eat are typically stripped of the fiber to be found in whole food.

Constipation, hiatus hernia, varicose veins and piles are rare in rural communities in the Third World. Cleave and a body of doctors with clinical experience, especially in Africa, state that the large quantities of whole starchy food eaten in the Third World allow food to pass more rapidly through the alimentary tract, giving the gut work it is designed to do, and leading to the formation of large soft stools.

By contrast, the constant straining caused by the bullet-like material formed from processed and concentrated starch and sugar is a direct cause of hernia, varicose veins and piles. Cleave goes further and proposes that the constant irritation, friction and pressure of constipation is a prime cause of more serious conditions, such as diverticular disease (a kind of rupture of the colon, common among middle-aged people in the Western World) and cancers of the large bowel and colon. Cleave states:

> The frequency of cancer increases steadily in each successive part of the colon, cancer of the rectum being one of the commonest in the body. It is significant that the irritant effect of any toxins on the intestinal wall must increase steadily in each of these successive parts, both on account of the actual greater production of toxins, and also on account of the progressive slowing that normally occurs in the colonic contents as they pass onwards.

In the nineteenth century it became understood that the irritants in soot caused skin cancer in chimney sweeps. In the last thirty years, we have recognized that the irritants in cigarette smoke cause cancers of the mouth, tongue, throat, bronchial passages and lungs of smokers. The proposal that processed sugars are a major cause of cancers of the lower gut has a similar basis—that the hard, toxic and offensive stools formed from sugars and other processed foods are a constant irritant to the gut, day after day, year after year.

The cause, or agent, of tooth decay is of course processed sugars. Almost all the qualified people who dispute this fact are either employees of the sugar industry or else funded by the sugar or food industries. Half a century ago the American dentist Weston Price spent nine years of his later life traveling the world, documenting the condition of teeth in many communities, for his book *Nutrition and Physical Degeneration*. In this epic work, he invariably found that when people ate traditional whole food, their teeth remained sound throughout life. He reinforced his point by examining the teeth of thousands of skeletons. He also found that when people started to eat Western food their teeth began to rot. Worse yet, as the title of his book indicates, he found that when parents switched from whole to processed food, the children born to them after the change frequently developed malformed teeth. When parents eat processed food, their children suffer.

SUGAR AND HEART DISEASE

Not only is the food we eat in the West heavy in processed sugars and starches. We also eat far too much animal fat. Animals today are bred to be fat, and we eat far more fatty meat than was eaten in our grandparents' day. Cheap foods such as sausages and beefburgers are made with masses of fatty waste from animal carcasses. We also consume a lot of full-fat dairy products such as milk, butter and cheese. And we eat quantities of fat made palatable by the addition of sugar in such things as chocolate and candy. How does all this affect the cardiovascular system?

Heart attacks and strokes are preceded by the buildup of certain types of fat in the blood, which in turn lead to the buildup of fatty deposits on the inside of blood vessels. Thus the blood vessels in the body, heart and brain begin to narrow. This process can be compared with the furring of domestic water pipes. High blood pressure ("hypertension") is a warning sign that the blood vessels are becoming silted up with fatty deposits ("atherosclerosis"). Eventually the vessels become so narrow that a blood clot ("thrombus") is liable to form. Should the clot block the blood vessels of the brain the result is a stroke ("cerebral thrombosis"). If the blood vessels of the heart are blocked the result is a heart attack ("coronary thrombosis").

Since around half the deaths in the United States today are caused by heart attacks and strokes, we have a powerful reason to find out what causes the buildup of fat in the blood and on the walls of blood vessels.

One cause of heart disease is bad blood—not, of course, in the sense that leads to knife fights in Sardinia, but in the sense of blood containing too much of the wrong type of blood fat. In particular, scientists have recently made a vital distinction between "high-density lipoprotein" and "low-density lipoprotein." It is now understood that the problem is not the volume of fat in the blood, but the type of fat in the blood. High-density lipoprotein (HDL), which is fat (lipid) bound up with protein, consists of tiny globules, which are, effectively, abrasive; one of its functions may be to scour the inside surfaces of blood vessels. Low-density lipoprotein, by contrast, consists of relatively large globules, and is sticky. Healthy blood has a high proportion of HDL. Unhealthy blood has a high proportion of LDL. LDL is behind the buildup of cholesterol in the blood, and high cholesterol levels are known to increase the risk of a heart attack. So, what causes a high proportion of LDL?

As soon as it became known that a major cause of heart disease is the buildup of certain types of fat in the blood, dietary fat became the popular villain. Nowadays people are liable to believe that eating fat is a bad idea because, well, fat is fat: we assume that fat in the blood (or, indeed, body fat) is made from the fats we eat from meat or dairy products, oils, cakes, cookies, chocolate, etc. In fact, though, the human body does not merely turn a dietary substance into its equivalent in the body.

Once upon a time athletic coaches thought that the only way to build up their champions was to feed them meat, because meat is animal muscle. So boxers and football stars were fed steaks. Actually, it is just as sensible to feed cereal to athletes; the body converts starch into energy for the muscles, and cereal also contains protein. Under a similar presumption, candy manufacturers sell their goods by associating processed sugars with blood sugar, suggesting that active children need candy bars; whereas, once again, whole cereals are a better source of energy.

In the case of fats, the story is not so simple. It is certain that we in the West eat far too much animal fat, notably in meat, in dairy products and in many convenience foods. And it is certain that animal fats, eaten in excess, are a prime cause of the buildup of fatty deposits on the walls of blood vessels. The next chapter ("Swallow It Whole") recommends that we eat much less fat, especially animal fat. At the same time, though, anything else we eat that causes an increase in the proportion of LDL in the blood will increase fat in the blood vessels and will therefore also increase the risk of a heart attack.

T. L. Cleave made a study of the risk of heart disease in the West and showed that, in country after country, the rise was preceded by an acceleration of processed sugar consumption. In Britain, for example, the great rise in sugar consumption occurred toward the end of the nineteenth century, and the great rise in heart disease started about twenty years later. In the early years of this century heart disease was uncommon.

Doctors who study the patterns of health and disease in populations are known as epidemiologists. (The word comes from the Greek *epi*, meaning "upon"; *demos,* meaning "people"; and *logos,* meaning "study"; so literally it means "those who study what comes upon the people." Hence, "epidemic.") In the case of sugar, epidemiologists have proposed the "Rule of Seventy and Twenty," which refers to the fact that various Western diseases, including heart disease and obesity, become epidemic around twenty years after a population starts to eat more than seventy pounds of processed sugar a year.

The Rule of Seventy and Twenty is an effective rule of thumb. Other Western diseases, notably of the stomach and gut, seem to take rather longer to develop. On the other hand, diabetes can develop with startling speed in populations introduced to sugar by Westernization. Their bodies have a low tolerance for processed sugar.

THE CLINICAL EVIDENCE

In the 1960s Professor John Yudkin fed high levels of processed sucrose to nineteen student volunteers in London and after some weeks found that the blood of some of his volunteers—who were eating around three times as much sugar as they would normally eat—had become stickier and fattier. He also found that there was more insulin in their blood, which increases the risk of diabetes and also of heart disease. A majority of the volunteers did not react in this way, which would indicate that only some of us are sensitive to processed sugar. Were it otherwise, we would all develop diabetes and have heart attacks.

Yudkin is a well-known campaigner against processed sugar. His experimental results and his views have always been vehemently attacked by the representatives and the supporters of the world sugar trade. It is now commonly assumed that Yudkin's results were suspect—"untypical," as scientists politely say. Yet in 1983, in his contribution to the book *Medical Applications of Clinical Nutrition,* Dr. Sheldon Reiser reviewed well over a hundred clinical studies, most of which supported Yudkin's work. These studies showed that when animals, or human volunteers, were fed high levels of sugars, the levels of insulin and low-density lipoprotein in the blood increased. Furthermore, when volunteers cut down or completely cut out their consumption of sugars, undesirable types of fats in the blood dropped. The results were found in a proportion of subjects, evidently those vulnerable to sugar. Reiser also noted that processed sugars and saturated fats seem to work together in combination.

The case against processed sugars is mounting. Meanwhile it is certain that nobody ever came to any harm from cutting sugars out, totally.

CONFUSION OR COVER-UP?

Food manufacturers, as well as sugar manufacturers and importers, are as reluctant to accept the dangers of processed sugar, as cigarette manufacturers are to accept that smoking is deadly. Indeed, the sugar problem is bigger than the tobacco problem because sugar is mixed into every kind of food.

The defenders of processed sugars have also made much of two potentially muddling issues. First, for many years food scientists made the disastrous mistake of grouping sugars and starches together as "carbohydrate" (the reason being that both sugars and starches supply energy to the body). Second, it still is not generally understood why processed sugars are bad for us, whereas the natural sugars in fruits and vegetables are good for us. What's the difference?

The body needs sugar for all its functions. Body sugar is made from carbohydrates; and starchy foods such as cereals, bread, pasta and certain vegetables are as good a source of sugar for the body as are sweet foods. A proper level of blood sugar is essential for physical and mental well-being, and a sandwich or plate of spaghetti a day does indeed help you work, rest and play.

So do the fruits and vegetables containing natural sugar. One of the lists at the end of this chapter (page 101) is of foods high in natural sugars, which are nutritious. They contain many vitamins and minerals, and also the fiber the body needs, as well as energy from sugars.

Processed sugars poison the body not because they are sugars but because they are processed, and therefore drained of nourishment. Why, then, do we eat them?

Professor Yudkin's answer, that sugars are "highly palatable," obviously has some truth in it. But why should the body accept the amount of sugars we eat, given that processed sugars have such disastrous effects on our health and well-being? The explanation that sugars are "highly palatable" seems thin. Another answer is that sugars are an excellent commodity—they are cheap, do not rot, are easily transported, heavily advertised and very profitable. But this explanation also seems inadequate; a product must be attractive in the first place before advertising will work. Sugar has a magnetism unique among all substances we eat and drink. What is it in processed sugars that overwhelms the body's defenses?

The answer begins to emerge when we delve into the

nature of the disease which, after tooth decay, is most un-
equivocally caused by processed sugars: adult-onset diabetes.

DIABETES: THE SUGAR DISEASE

Thomas Willis, the seventeenth-century doctor who first
identified diabetes after noting the sweet-smelling urine of his
rich patients, wrote in 1685, in Latin, "I do much disapprove
things preserved or very much sweetened with sugar." Intu-
itively realizing that food containing energy but no nourishment can cause vitamin-deficiency diseases, he added, "I
judge the invention of it and its immoderate use to have very
much contributed to the vast increase of scurvy in this last
age."

Dr. Willis waited before publishing his news. He had
been court physician to King Charles II, who had enjoyed
the revenue from the slave trade and so from processed
sugar. It would not have been tactful for Willis to press his
point. And from that day to this, many well-placed doctors,
including a few who are consultants to the food industry,
have minced their words about the relationship between processed foods and disease.

Word about the connection between processed sugars
and diabetes is, however, getting out, in large part because
the epidemiological evidence is now very strong. In the 1980
report on dietary fiber, the Royal College of Physicians
noted:

> A high prevalence of diabetes seems to be charac-
> teristic of recently urbanized populations. Exam-
> ples are Indians and Zulus in South Africa, Yemeni
> Jews in Israel, American Indians throughout the
> United States, Maoris in New Zealand, and Polyne-
> sians in the Central Pacific island of Nauru. The
> dietary change which has most often been blamed
> has been the adoption of refined sugar.

The exploitation of phosphates to be found on Nauru has
brought the islanders the highest per capita income in the

world, but at the price of their health. Dr. Denis Burkitt has told me that the incidence of diabetes on Nauru has been estimated at 42 percent. But when Alexander Frater visited the island for the *Observer* in October 1982, a European nurse there told him that the incidence was 90 percent. Dr. Thoma, head of medical services, said to Frater:

> We have the second highest rate of diabetes in the world, after the Pima Indians of Phoenix, Arizona. The disease can be prevented and controlled by diet. People here eat too much, and the food is all canned and refined.

The Canadian Dr. Frederick Banting, who isolated insulin in the 1920s, had little doubt about the cause of diabetes in adults. His own observations told Banting that natural sugar is a food but processed sugar is a poison. In 1924 he visited Panama and spoke to a doctor examining men applying for work on the Panama Canal, who had found that none of them had diabetes. Banting commented:

> This is the more remarkable because a large percentage of the labourers were natives of Dominica, where a main article of diet was sugar-cane. From the time the children are weaned until they die they eat the sugar-cane. There are also wealthy Spaniards who live in Panama who eat large quantities of refined cane sugar. Indeed much of their food is cooked in syrup. The incidence of diabetes amongst this class is surprisingly high.

Food containing sugars in a natural state—bananas, oranges, apples, grapes and other fruits, sweet potato, onions, carrots and other vegetables, and the cane and beet from which sugar is processed—are nutritious and good for us. The cause of diabetes is not sugar, but sugar in an intensely concentrated form. Diabetes could theoretically develop from eating massive amounts of honey, which is sugar refined by bees, or dried fruits such as dates, raisins, and currants. But we are satisfied by small amounts of these foods, which are to be avoided only by diabetics. Also, honey and dried fruits are nutritious.

So how is diabetes caused? Our good health and sense of well-being depend on the level of sugar in our blood being neither too high nor too low. Hunger is triggered when the level of sugar in the blood falls below a certain point. Starches and sugars, when eaten, both raise blood sugar levels. Starches, eaten in the form of cereals, bread or pasta, or potatoes, say, raise the blood sugar at a natural speed, as do the sugars in fruit and vegetables which seep into the bloodstream. The sense of fullness and satisfaction derived from eating such foods is reliable, especially when the flour in bread or in the pasta is whole-wheat (and therefore not robbed of fiber, vitamins and minerals).

But because of its concentration, processed sugar shoots into the bloodstream and is liable to raise the blood sugar level too high. The immediate effect of this sugar rush is very pleasant. But after a certain point, eating sugar becomes nauseating. This is especially noticeable if the initial blood sugar level is very low, as it is in a dieter or in a runner after a long-distance race; both feel the need for sugar but can suffer if they eat a candy bar rather than fruit or a sandwich.

When the level of blood sugar gets too high, the body lowers it by releasing insulin from the pancreas into the bloodstream. The faster the blood sugar level rises, and the higher it goes, the more intense and sudden the reaction of the pancreas. This "panic" reaction results in too much insulin pouring into the bloodstream, so that, paradoxically, the result of eating or drinking food saturated with processed sugars is to change the blood sugar level from too high to too low. Medically this phenomenon is known as "rebound hypoglycemia."

THE "ASLEEP AT THE WHEEL" SYNDROME

In due course this oversensitization of the pancreas is liable to lead to a condition which can be termed "hyperinsulinism" or "hypoglycemia," a doctor's term for the whiplash effect of eating and drinking refined sugars (or alcoholic drinks, which have the same result). Hypoglycemia has achieved a certain vogue recently, partly because Richard Harris and Julie Andrews have both revealed that they are sufferers, because of alcohol and sweets respectively. As Julie Andrews confessed to *Woman* magazine: "If I made the foolish mistake of having a brownie when I thought I was going to have an easy day and could indulge myself, I had the most awful fatigue and dizziness. You wouldn't believe it."

This state can be dangerous. The one time I fell asleep at the wheel was after running a half-marathon on a hot day, after which I ate two "Marathon" candy bars, which the race organizers had supplied to the runners. (This was before I had done the research for this book!) Half an hour after the race I was driving home, fast, down a motorway, and without any warning fell unconscious, and was jerked awake only by my head hitting the steering wheel.

In their processed form, sugars have the paradoxical effect of lowering blood sugar levels and setting up a need for the very food that converts quickly into blood sugar—that is, processed sugars. The dependency thus set up drives out the natural desire for starchy and sweet whole foods that supply blood sugar at a natural rate, because that rate comes to feel too slow. The body of someone who eats an average amount of processed sugars is liable to alternate between being too high in blood-sugar to being too low. Balance is destroyed. The natural patterns of mood, emotion, sleep, energy and fatigue, concentration and reverie are invaded and confused.

Sugar is with us all the time. It is a term of endearment. It is a comfort.

> The habit of eating for pleasure or comfort such high energy foods as sweets, chocolates, cakes, biscuits and desserts is initiated in childhood. These items may be given out for good behaviour, and withheld as punishment,

points out the Royal College of Physicians' report on obesity; which goes on to suggest, reasonably enough, that, so trained, adults will turn to such foods when anxious or depressed.

Sugar is one of the things "little girls are made of." Babies are kept quiet by sweet water rubbed on their pacifiers. The newborn infant prefers sugar solution to water. Children so small that they cannot see over the counter beg for candy, and chocolates are a conventional gift to a loved one. In service stations, newspaper shops, supermarket checkouts, candy is the impulse buy. In Britain the last course at table or in a restaurant, the naughty temptation, is called "the sweet." On average, everyone in the United States eats a ton of processed sugars every twenty years. How is it that a food so common and so attractive can be so bad for us?

WHY SUGAR MAKES YOU FAT—AND WORSE

Together with alcohol, processed sugars have a special quality that causes the sugar eater to gain fat. Discussions of energy balance tend to treat it like a bank balance: put too much energy in and you get fat, put less energy in and you get thin. People who defend sugar always make a lot of this idea, pointing out that carbohydrates, including sugar, have an energy value of 3.75 per unit of weight compared with 4.1 for protein and the much higher figure of 9.3 for fat (the figures are often quoted as 4:4:9, but these are more precise). The boldest defenders of processed sugar go so far as to suggest that sugar is therefore a low-energy food and an essential part of any weight-reducing regime! In Washington, the White House is surrounded by the headquarters of sugar and processed food lobbyists, who try to sell this notion to legislators.

Even if you accept the metaphor that the body is a bank, this argument is specious. Foods containing sugar are indeed low-energy foods—when they are whole foods, whose natural sugars are bound up with fiber, and with other nutrients, and water. A pound of apples, for example, has an energy content of around 175 calories; a pound of grapes, 225 to 275 calories. Apples include around 12 percent natural sugar, grapes, around 13 to 16 percent natural sugar. Four ounces of candy, by comparison, amount to 300 to 500 calories. Candy is little more than processed sugars; some, like toffee, have added fats. And as well as being nourishing, apples and grapes will be more satisfying than candy, simply because of their bulk: they are more filling. It is only when sugars occur naturally in whole foods that they can honestly be described as "low-energy."

Processed sugars are not, of course, the only thing we eat that can make us fat. Since the turn of this century, the amount of dietary fats people in Western countries eat, expressed as a percentage of total calories consumed, has increased from 30 percent to around 40 to 42 percent. One major reason why we eat more fat is that food manufacturers make fats palatable by mixing them with processed sugars— for example, chocolate bars, ice cream, cakes and cookies. Eat less processed sugars and you are very likely indeed to eat less fats.

But the human body is not just a piggy bank for food. The body reacts to different types of food in different ways. In particular, any food that has the effect of overstimulating a healthy pancreas will tend to make you fat for reasons which have nothing to do with the energy content of the food. The reason is as follows. The insulin poured into the bloodstream as a result of overstimulation of the pancreas does not merely "dissolve" the blood sugar, as some books suggest. The story does not end there. The insulin gets rid of the blood sugar by a process that, first, converts the blood sugar into low-density lipoprotein, the type of blood fat that is implicated in heart disease; and then it dumps this fat into the store of fatty tissue.

This is why concentrated sugars have a fundamentally different effect on the body than sugars in fruit. The higher the concentration of processed sugars in food, the greater the impact on the pancreas. Soft drinks like colas are an example, because the water with which the sugars in soft drinks are diluted does not have a protective effect. Chocolate and candy bars, which are more than half processed sugars, mixed with fats, are also liable to overstimulate the pancreas and so make you doubly fat.

WHY CHILDREN SHOULD NOT EAT CANDY

Vigorously active people can consume processed sugars and not get fat, for reasons touched on in the last chapter, and enlarged upon in Chapter 5 ("More Air! More Air!"). If muscle tissue or the liver is low in glycogen, then the insulin released by the pancreas will convert blood sugar into glycogen. Because glycogen in the body is bound up with water, a post-diet "binge" on sweet things adds water to the body too—which is why it has such a dramatic effect on body weight.

There again, people who run a lot, as children naturally do, or who engage in a lot of sport, as children ordinarily do, are using the glycogen in their muscles all the time. So a cola drink or a candy bar is liable to be converted not into body fat, but into muscle glycogen. Only active people can efficiently use processed sugars as body fuel. This does not mean—whatever the soft-drink and candy manufacturers may tell you—that the body of an active person has any *need* for processed sugars. Starchy foods convert just as readily into glycogen.

Besides, "hits" from processed sugars abuse the pancreas of active and sedentary people alike. Mothers who want to ensure that their children do not become diabetic in later life should feed them plenty of whole-meal bread, with sugar-free spreads. (There is also reason to believe that constant overstimulation of any gland, of which the pancreas is one, becomes addictive in time, and that people who, when children, consume a lot of processed sugars are liable when adult to turn to alcohol, which has the same effect on the pancreas. The child's candy becomes the adult's martini.)

OVERWEIGHT AND DIABETES

Medical textbooks tend to associate diabetes with obesity. In this, they are misleading. Obesity is, rather, fairly likely to be a signal of a prediabetic state, hypoglycemia, in which an abused pancreas is nevertheless still capable of overreacting to the processed sugar "rush." A hypoglycemic person is particularly liable to gain fat, and therefore particularly likely to try one futile diet regime after another. Sad to say, the weight problem of a hypoglycemic person is liable to be eased only by the onset of diabetes. Diabetes in adults is caused by an abused pancreas eventually becoming exhausted. Then the process whereby insulin converts sugar to fat in the blood, and hence to fat in the body, ceases. Instead, the blood sugar is, first, dumped into the kidneys, and then into the urine, and thereafter builds up to dangerous levels which are deadly unless checked.

It follows, therefore, that a rather sudden weight loss, especially in adults in their forties or fifties who had previously been gaining weight, is a signal that a prediabetic state has become clinical diabetes.

Professor Harry Keen of Guys Hospital in London is a leading specialist who is disinclined to agree that sugar is to blame for diabetes. Nevertheless, in 1975 he published a highly significant study. He asked 711 people diagnosed as diabetic to recall their heaviest weight in the past, and also weighed them. He repeated the process with relatives of the diabetics, and with a "control" group of unrelated non-diabetics. He found that the weight of the diabetics was much the same as that of the other people. The one outstanding finding was that on average, the diabetics had weighed 20 pounds more before being diagnosed as diabetic. That is to say, these people, prediabetic, were on average 20 pounds heavier than they were when clinically diabetic.

Processed sugars make you fat, for three reasons. First, they contain no nourishment and therefore cheat the body's natural desire for nourishment. Second, because they are concentrated and heavy in calories, they deceive the appetite. Calorie for calorie, the appetite is better satisfied by whole food, which is bulky. Third, and most important, processed sugars make you fat because they disturb the insulin hormone. Processed sugars are the link between obesity, diabetes and heart disease.

Sedentary people who eat an average amount of processed sugars (or who drink a lot of alcohol) face one of two dismal futures. Either they will eat enough nutritious food, plus the sugar, in which case they will end up overweight or even obese, and by middle age be at risk of diabetes, heart disease or other Western diseases. Or they will avoid gaining weight in the only way sedentary people can, by eating half or maybe even less of the nourishing food their bodies need, in which case the result will be malaise, debilitation, and eventually chronic deficiency states—the junk-food syndrome.

SUGAR ADDICTION

If processed sugars were unknown and were now introduced, and their effects observed, they would be made illegal. We shy away from the word "addictive," tending to apply it only to substances which, as well as being poisonous, are illegal. But, after all, it was only 200 years ago that mothers quieted their babies by means of opium smeared on a little finger. Later, opium became illegal.

We crave sugar. That should be clue enough. We speak jokingly of being "sugar junkies" and wanting a "sugar hit," and jokes are always clues. A substance is addictive when it drives out a natural body function, replacing it with an artificial function on which the body then comes to depend. Smoking, for example, is addictive for two separate reasons. The carbon monoxide in tobacco smoke inhibits the flow of oxygen to the blood, and the nicotine in tobacco inhibits the flow of hormones known as endorphins, the body's natural painkillers. The craving for cigarettes after giving up smoking is not "just in the mind"; the body learns to crave carbon monoxide and nicotine.

In the same way, processed sugars overwhelm the body's natural desire for the sugar within fruit or the starch in vegetables and cereals. Eating processed sugars causes an artificially high blood sugar level; then, because of the body's defense system, an artificially low blood sugar level; and so a craving for sugar. As Mr. Mars discovered, eating one Mars Bar creates the desire for another Mars Bar.

SUGARS IN FOOD

It is not easy to avoid eating processed sugars. The following table is designed to help you. The first list itemizes foods heavy in processed sugars. It begins with foods that contain more than 40 percent processed sugars. These are mostly cakes and candy, but many sweet breakfast cereals are saturated with processed sugars and are often high in salt as well. The middle part of the list, of foods containing more than 15 percent sugars, includes some items tasting fairly savory or thought of as "health" foods, such as relishes and flavored yogurt. Note the fruit salads, which are between 15 and 25 percent sugar when canned in syrup. Note also Coca-Cola, Pepsi-Cola and other cola drinks, which are around 10 percent sugars by weight, but whose calories are 100 percent supplied by sugars.

Almost all canned food has added sugars. Look at the ingredients label for sugars in their various forms, and remember that many food manufacturers are not as open as they might be about the amount of sugars their products contain. There is no law obliging all manufacturers to state the total percentage of all sugars in processed food—there should be such a law.

The second list is of foods high in naturally occurring sugars which also contain many nutrients. While honey and dried fruit are both nutritious, it is best to eat them sparingly. Fruit juice has more sugar than the fruit itself, the fibrous content having been removed; prefer the whole fruit.

The body needs sugar for energy, but you do not need to eat food containing sugars. This is because starches convert to sugar in the body, just as readily as dietary sugars. The third list is designed to wean you off processed sugars: it is a selection of cereals, vegetables and fruits containing little or no sugar, together with other foods—meat and dairy products, for example—that are low in sugars but on the other hand high in fats.

The processed foods always to avoid are sweets and sweet fats, and processed cereals and vegetables to which sugars, fats or salt have been added. These have little nour-

TABLE 1: SUGARS IN FOOD

Foods High in Processed Sugars

	Percent of weight		Percent of weight
Sugar (white)	100	Fruit salad (canned)[2]	25
Sugar (brown)	100	Jello	25
Meringues	95	Butter cookies[1]	25
Water ice	95	Tomato ketchup[1]	23
Hard candies	88	Dairy ice cream[1]	23
Chocolate chip cookies[1]	75	100 percent Bran cereal	22
Drinking chocolate (dry)	74	Peaches (canned in syrup)[1,2]	20
Milky Way	73	Fruit-flavor yogurt[2]	18
Chewing gum	72	All-Bran	15
Toffees	70	Mayonnaise[1]	15
Jam[2]	69	Doughnuts	15
Marmalade[2]	69	Plain cookies[1]	15
Chocolate (plain)	60	Coca-Cola	10
Chocolate (milk)	57	Pepsi-Cola	10
Sugar Smacks	56	Canned sweet corn[2]	9
Bounty bar	54	Rice Krispies	8
Apple Jacks	52	Special K	8
Rich fruit cake[1,2]	50	Wheaties	8
Fruit Loops	49	Corn Flakes	7
Chocolate cookies[1]	45	Peanut butter[1]	7
Sugar Frosted Flakes	39	Grape-Nuts	7
Cheesecake (fruit flavor)[1]	36	Diet bread	7
Sweet relish[1]	35	Orange drink (dilute)	6
Cap'n Crunch	32	Lemon drink (dilute)	6
Raisin Bran[2]	30	Canned beans[1,2]	5

1. Varies with brand, but usually not greatly.
2. Including some natural sugars content.

Foods High in Natural Sugars			
	Percent		Percent
Honey[1]	76	Figs (fresh)	10
Raisins	68	Orange juice	10
Dated (dried)	66	Sweet potato	
Currants	63	(boiled)	9
Figs (dried)	53	Peaches	9
Milk (skimmed,		Oranges[3]	9
dried)[2]	53	Spring onions	9
Apricots (dried)	43	Damsons	
Prunes (dried)	40	(stewed)	8
Milk (dried)[2]	39	Tangerines	8
Prunes (stewed)	20	Horseradish	
Bananas	16	(raw)	7
Lychees (raw)	16	Chestnuts	7
Grapes, white[3]	16	Apricots (raw)	7
Mangoes	15	Blackcurrants	7
Grapes, black[3]	15	Coconut	
Apple juice	13	(desiccated)	6
Nectarines	12	Blackberries	6
Cherries	12	Strawberries	6
Apples (raw)[3]	12	Passion fruit	6
Greengage		Apricots	
plums	12	(stewed)	6
Pineapple[3]	12	Raspberries	6
Pomegranates		Carrots	5
(juice)	12	Grapefruit[3]	5
Pears[3]	11	Melons	5
Onions (fried)	10	Onions	5
Beetroot		Chick peas	5
(cooked)	10	Plums	
Damson plums	10	(stewed)	5

1. Honey has nutrients but in a sense is refined (by bees).
2. Lactose.
3. Juice from these fruits has 1 to 2 percent more sugar.

Foods Low in Sugars

	Percent		Percent
Fresh milk[1]	5	Avocado pears	2
Natural yogurt[1]	5	Cucumbers	2
Leeks (boiled)	5	Corn on the cob	2
Almonds	4	Brussels sprouts	2
Carrots (boiled)	4	Puffed wheat	2
Coconut	4	Beans	1
Peas (canned)[2]	4	Peas	1
Loganberries	3	Squash	1
Tomato juice	3	Lettuce	1
Lemons	3	Spinach	1
Nuts	3	Celery	1
Eggplant	3	Cauliflower	1
Gooseberries		Lentils	1
(stewed)	3	Spaghetti,	
Tomatoes	3	pastas	1
Parsnips (boiled)	3	Potatoes	1
Tomato soup[2]	3	Watercress	1
Vegetable soup[2]	3	Shredded wheat	1
Water biscuits	2	Olives	Trace
Instant potato[2]	2	Rice	Trace
White cabbage		Porridge	Trace
(boiled)	2	Tea	Trace
Cheese[1]	2	Mushrooms	0
White bread,		Meat, poultry	0
rolls[2]	2	Fish	0
Wholemeal		No-cal drinks	0
bread[2]	2	Water,	
Peas (fresh)	2	mineral water	0

1. Lactose. Yogurt also has a little galactose.
2. Processed sugars.

Chief source of information: *McCance and Widdowson's The Composition of Foods* edited by A. A. Paul and D. A. T. Southgate (HMSO 1978); also *Composition of Foods* (Agriculture Handbook No. 8, USDA).

ishment compared with whole fresh food, and often contain cocktails of additives. By contrast, the fruit and some vegetables that are rich in natural sugars are good for you almost however much of them you eat. By themselves fruit and vegetables cannot make you fat; it is only the addition of fats (in the form of cream to fruit or fats and oil to vegetables) and sugars (as in syrups added to canned fruit) that is fattening. Fruit and vegetables are most nourishing when eaten raw.

4

Swallow It Whole

The word "health" in English is based on an Anglo-Saxon word "hale" meaning "whole": that is, to be healthy is to be whole. Likewise, the English "holy" is based on the same root as "whole." All of this indicates that man has sensed always that wholeness or integrity is an absolute necessity to make life worth living.

> —David Bohm
> *Wholeness and the Implicate Order*

We always had plenty, our children never cried from hunger, neither were our people in want. The rapids of Rock River furnished us with an abundance of excellent fish, and the land being very fertile never failed to produce good crops of corn, beans, pumpkins, and squashes. If a prophet had come to our village in those days and told us that the things were to take place which have since come to pass, none of our people would have believed him.

> —Black Hawk, Chief of the Souk and Fox
> In *Touch the Earth,* by T. C. McLuhan

MORE DIETING MEMOIRS

In my dieting days, I carried around a leaflet called the "Unit Eating Guide" whose introduction promised:

> An evolutionary approach . . . to the problem of correct eating. No longer will you be able to say you feel hungry. This is because a very wide variety of foods can be freely taken at any time.

Ah! Magic! A diet that didn't involve cutting calories! No wonder I picked it up. The principle of this system was to fasten the mind of the dieter on the monster, carbohydrate: "Keep your carbohydrate consumption down to a low level by taking little of the carbohydrate foods, but as much as you like of the noncarbohydrate foods."

It was a handy little guide, it listed food in three groups. Group A was "eat as much as you like." It included:

Duck	Processed cheese
Lard	Cream
Liver paste	Margarine
Tripe	Cooking Oil
Cod	Salad oil
Flathead	Cabbage
Leather jacket	Okra
Oysters	Olives
Pollack	Pumpkin
Snails	Zucchini
Butter	Ginger
Cream cheese	Gravy

Comfortingly, the guide described this list as "quite straight-forward ordinary foods, and you can eat them whenever you like."

Group C was printed on red paper. "Danger! Avoid if possible!" was printed on top of this list, rather like the road signs that warn you of falling rocks. Looking at the leaflet now, I well recall the feelings I had as I peered down the list of foods which I thought were making me into Michelin Man. They included:

Ale	Ice cream
All-Bran	Macaroni
Bread, brown	Oatmeal
Bread, white	Port
Bun	Potato
Cereals	Spaghetti
Chocolate	Sugar
Flour	Taro
Fructose	Teff
Gin	Toffees
Grapes	Vermicelli
Honey	Yam

There was a time when I knew these lists more or less by heart. Meals of syrup, toffees, tonic water, and vermicelli were Out. Menus of garfish, grouper, gurnet and haddock were In; as were snapper, seaslugs, shrimps and skate, or mayonnaise, mustard, pepper and pickles. I wondered, eyeing the oysters in the fish store, which fish was the leather jacket. I believed that if, in a café, I was told, "Sorry, we're out of taro and teff," I was missing nothing that would do me any good. The introduction warned against the foods in group C because these were, it said, "foods that are rich in carbohydrate, and don't contain much in the way of nutrients." The guide was put out in 1972.

THE CONFUSION OF STARCH WITH SUGAR

Dr. Irwin Stillman's *Doctor's Quick Weight Loss Diet* was popular at about the same time. One of his diets goes as follows: "The usual basic restriction at its strongest may be summed up in one sentence: don't touch carbohydrates, sugar, salt, fruits, cereals, bread, rice, potatoes, alcohol."

Don't touch! In a like vein, Richard Mackarness, a psychiatrist, wrote *Eat Fat and Grow Slim,* which, its publishers claim, has sold over a million copies. While warning against sugar and refined foods, Mackarness says:

> Try to develop a carbohydrate alarm system, so that whenever you are confronted with a food which does or even *might* contain carbohydrate, a little bell goes off in your head and you avoid the temptation to eat it.

"The first thing to realize," writes Dr. Mackarness, "is that it is carbohydrate (starch and sugar) and carbohydrate only, which fattens fat people."

The British Consumers' Association is also enthusiastic about low-carbohydrate diets, as an alternative to diets that cut calories. In *Which? Way to Slim,* published in 1978, the authors say:

> The foods which are richest in carbohydrates are, on the whole, the ones which are poorest in proteins, vitamins and minerals. . . . The low carbohydrate diet is therefore particularly suitable for growing children.

Much like my "Unit Eating Guide" and Dr. Mackarness, *Which?* says of carbohydrate-rich food: "Think of it as a traffic light. The red light means STOP for the things to avoid. . . ." And the list includes bread, breakfast cereals, cookies, flour, honey, nuts, potatoes, spaghetti, sugar and sweets. The basic message is that the baddies are sugar and starch, lumped together as carbohydrates.

Vogue magazine has followed a similar policy for many years. In the 1960s it said: "The simplest do-it-yourself answer is—we're sorry to say—some kind of crash diet. It's human nature to want quick results, so, for quick returns, cut out starch and sugar."

In 1966 *Vogue* produced a Peanut Diet, "devised by a leading nutrition consultant." "Forbidden foods include everything made with flour or cornflour, root vegetables, peas, beans, cereals, pastas, all sugar, sweets, sweetened drinks." The dieter is told to replace one of the main meals of the day with 2 ounces of peanuts (with salt) and also an orange.

The Vogue Book of Diets and Exercise, published in 1980, lists various low-carbohydrate diets, including one recommended by Edgar S. Gordon, Professor of Medicine at the University of Wisconsin; one created for the late Aga Khan (a man not noted for a slim figure); and one by Robert Atkins, of *Dr. Atkins' Diet Revolution* and *Dr. Atkins' Nutrition Breakthrough.* No peanuts, says Dr. Atkins. And, in the Jovian style he shares with Dr. Stillman, Dr. Tarnower and all the most effective snake-oil salesmen—prophetic, fatherly, threatening—he says:

> Super Don'ts. Put these out of your life (and your recipes). Bread, cereal, corn, ice cream, ketchup, macaroni, milk, potatoes, pulse vegetables, rice, spaghetti, sugar, sweets, chewing gum, water biscuits. Note: one piece of chewing gum can spoil the whole chemical balance.

Everybody who has been on a low-carbohydrate diet will recognize the language used to make the dieter conform. "Danger!" "Try to develop a carbohydrate alarm system." "Think of it as a traffic light." ". . . the whole chemical balance." "Should be taken only sparingly." The metaphors and images buzz around the brain of the bemused dieter, who is invited to think of carbohydrates as an abyss, a burglar, oncoming traffic, a toxin, or a medicine. Always the dieter is told to distrust his or her own body.

Until Audrey Eyton's *F-Plan Diet,* the best-selling diet book in Britain was Professor John Yudkin's *This Slimming Business,* first published in 1958. Yudkin is best known professionally for his hostility to processed sugars. But in his writings for the general public, dieters in particular, this hostility extended to all carbohydrates. As a nutrition consultant and author and writer of numerous articles (sometimes under a *nom de plume*) he probably did more than any other nutritionist to have Britons believe that for the dieter, carbohydrates are the villain.

Yudkin's theory of nutrition is that the food eaten by our hunter-gatherer ancestors was meat, fish, roots, berries, fruit and leaves, that it was rich in protein and also fat, but included little carbohydrate. On this theory, he gives us a

"Stone Age Diet" to follow: "The nearer we get to man's hunting and food gathering diet, the more likely we are to be well-nourished, and the more we can depend on our instinctive choice." Yudkin sees agriculture as a snare. In his view, the discovery of cereals encouraged settlement and the beginning of civilization. The agriculturist's food, composed chiefly of carbohydrate, contains less protein and fat than that of the hunter-gatherer. Yudkin concludes, in a passage which in effect provides the intellectual underpinning for all low-carbohydrate diets, "My theory is that this is the fundamental fault with the diets of civilization." He then goes on to set out his system of "carbohydrate units," explaining that all the dieter need do is memorize a long list of carbohydrate-rich foods and, on the whole, avoid them.

THE POWER OF THE SUGAR INDUSTRY

Not so much is heard nowadays of low-carbohydrate diets. One reason is that late in his career Yudkin changed his view, and came to acknowledge that starch should not be confused with sugar.

Unfortunately, a powerful section of industry still prefers to confuse the issue. In England the Health Education Council commissioned a report on the information the British public receives about sugar, then suppressed this report after pressure was applied by representatives of the sugar industry. The report, *Sweet Nothings,* shows that the British public is still receiving conflicting advice about starch and sugar. For example, the British Medical Association's *You and Your Baby,* produced for mothers in 1977, says: "Do eat sensibly. It means eating little carbohydrate." Another leaflet, produced for expectant mothers in 1975, says: "Potatoes, bread, sugar, cakes and biscuits are carbohydrates. They provide energy and warmth, but should only be taken sparingly."

Keeping Fit in Retirement, a publication produced by the National Dairy Council, says: "If you want to lose some weight, cut out or reduce some of the 'starchy' foods you eat. These are bread, cakes, pastry, sugar, jam, rice, biscuits, cereals and potatoes."

Ironically, given Yudkin's hostility to processed sugar, his old argument that starch and sugar are equally objectionable is turned on its head by the sugar manufacturers, who argue that sugar and starch are equally desirable. The British Sugar Bureau, a publicity organization for sugar manufacturers, published *Questions and Answers on Sugar* in 1977, circulating it free to doctors, surgeons, health education officers, registered dietitians and the press. I first came across it on the shelves of the Health Education Council's library. *Questions and Answers* says that processed sugar is a

> carbohydrate which is easily absorbed and enables the body to replace lost energy quickly. This property is appreciated by athletes, sportsmen, busy mothers and active growing children. . . . Our calorie needs are provided by balanced meals containing protein, carbohydrates, including starches and sugars, and fats. When weight reduction is indicated most dietitians support an overall reduction of food intake.

In 1983 the British Sugar Bureau was at it again, this time circulating a new document, *Sweet Reason,* to doctors, dentists and health professionals. Sugar, says the industry, is good for hiccups and sealing wounds, and:

> A Scottish pharmacist reports successful treatment of varicose ulcers and severe bedsores with a mixture of granulated sugar, povidone iodine ointment and povidone iodine solution.

We would all be in better shape if the only thing we used sugar for is healing bedsores.

In the United States, Professor Frederick Stare, who has been Professor of Nutrition at the Harvard School of Public Health, has constantly spoken out in favor of sugar. "Most people could healthily double their sugar intake daily," he once said. His views have been very widely publicized by the sugar industry. Indeed, Dr. Stare is a good friend of the industry.

When housewives were asked in a survey to name the

foods that should be avoided when dieting, the eight foods most often named were:

Potatoes	62%
Bread	55%
Sugar	31%
Cakes	25%
Starches	22%
Sweets	16%
Fat	10%
Carbohydrate	7%

Cookies, pastry, fried food and butter came farther down the list. In the minds of dieters and would-be dieters, sugars and starches are mingled together. For the last twenty years and more, mothers, children, dieters, pensioners, physicians, dietitians, nutritionists, health educators, nurses, journalists and readers of newspapers have been taught to think of carbohydrates as bad food and to think of sugars and starches therefore as equally bad, or, if susceptible to the publicity of the sugar industry, as equally good.

THE MEDICAL REVOLUTION FOR THE 1980s

All this is changing now, and the change is radical. In February 1977 a committee of the United States Senate, chaired by Senator George McGovern, published a report, *Dietary Goals for the United States*. Senator McGovern's preliminary statement set the tone of a report which, more than any other single influence, is changing the food habits of Americans:

> The simple fact is that our diets have changed radically within the last fifty years, with great and often very harmful effects on our health. . . . Too much fat, too much sugar or salt, can be and are linked directly to heart disease, cancer, obesity and stroke, among other killer diseases. In all, six of the ten leading causes of death in the United States have

been linked to our diet. Those of us within Government have an obligation to acknowledge this.

The report begins by making the sharpest possible distinction between starch and sugar. It points out that processed foods saturated with sugar, fat and salt are massively advertised, whereas foods rich in starch—whole grains and vegetables—are rarely advertised. In less than thirty years, the consumption of grain, vegetables and fruits has dropped dramatically.

The report goes on to point out that starchy foods like cereals and vegetables are rich in vitamins and minerals (micronutrients), as is fruit:

> Increased consumption of fruit, vegetables and whole grains is also important with respect to supplying adequate amounts of micronutrients, vitamins and minerals. This is particularly important for those who are limiting their food intake to control weight or save money. For many people consumption may be reaching a critical level below which it may be difficult to obtain adequate levels of micronutrients.

Suddenly, in America, the doctors and scientists who knew the vital importance of whole food, and knew what was wrong with sugar, fat and salt, were no longer lonely voices: they had the American government behind them. *Dietary Goals* proposed that consumption of starchy foods (including naturally occurring sugars) be almost doubled (from a figure of 28 percent of total energy intake to 48 percent) and that the consumption of processed sugars be sharply cut (from 18 percent of energy intake to 10 percent):

	Total energy intake	
	U.S. 1977 (%)	*McGovern goal (%)*
Protein	12	12
Fats	42	30
Starches, etc.	28	48
Sugars	18	10
Total	100	100

The report also emphasizes that, completely contrary to what has been stated in so many dieting books, starchy foods are not fattening. Earlier in this book the twenty-three young men of Galway who lost weight on Dr. Denis Burkitt's potato diet were mentioned. The McGovern report points out that bread, too, is not fattening. Quite the reverse:

> Contrary to what most people think, bread in large amounts is an ideal food in a weight reducing program. . . . Slightly overweight young men lost weight in a painless and practically effortless manner when they included twelve slices of bread a day in their program. The bread was eaten with their meals. As a result, they became satiated before they consumed their usual quota of calories.

The young men were asked to go easy on sugars and fats; otherwise, they could eat what they liked—provided that they ate the bread. In eight weeks they had lost an average of over 12 pounds.

In 1983 the Royal College of Physicians of London, in its report on obesity, likewise made a clear distinction between starches and sugar, and also emphasized that starchy foods are not fattening:

> The public and many in the medical profession have come to consider dietary carbohydrates as being particularly conducive to weight gain and the development of obesity, no distinction being made between sucrose (sugar) and starch as sources of dietary carbohydrate.

And, referring to starches, the report went on to say that "low carbohydrate diets are inappropriate on general nutritional grounds."

The Royal College agrees with the McGovern committee that fats intake should be reduced to 30 percent of total calories. With processed sugar it goes a little further, recommending that we should eat half the amount we now eat.

In the last decade or so, countries all over the developed

world have been issuing recommendations along the same lines.

Between now and the end of the century, we may experience an enormous change in the practice of Western medicine: a move toward prevention. This movement will be encouraged by citizens who are appalled by the effects of drugs and who, by taking responsibility for themselves, will encourage doctors to practice the medicine of health rather than of illness. It will require massive reallocations of money; it is estimated that less than 1 percent of total health expenditure in America is devoted to the prevention of disease. And above all, it will require government and industry to work together with a will. Senator Charles Percy of the McGovern committee had this to say:

> Without government and industry commitment to good nutrition, the American people will continue to eat themselves to bad health. . . . Our national health depends on how well and how quickly government and industry respond.

WHOLE FOOD: THE FOUNDING DOCTORS

The story behind this radical new view of the relationship between the food we eat and obesity, health and disease begins with a group of British doctors who are having the impact on medicine that Darwin had on science and Keynes had on economics. These doctors, with their followers in America and other countries, have demonstrated beyond all reasonable doubt that the diseases that most of us suffer and die from in the West (and that are—often ineffectively— treated by the medicine of drugs and surgery) are caused, above all, by what we eat and what we do not eat. These noninfectious Western diseases can, therefore, be prevented.

So far the thesis of this book could be said to amount to two "don'ts." If you want to lose fat, and if you want to gain health, do not go on a diet, and do not eat processed foods, especially sugars. The rest of this chapter is concerned with good food—with the unprocessed whole cereals, vegetables and other fresh foods so long wrongly blamed as a cause of fatness, so long condemned as having little nourishment, now rightly championed as the staff of life.

T. L. Cleave has a reputation as the doctor who exposed the role of processed sugars in obesity and disease. But Cleave always, at the same time, advocated whole foods. He was opposed to the spoonful of sugar; he was in favor of the apple:

> It is perfectly true that calories in, for example, an apple are much the same as those in a teaspoon of sugar, and therefore at first sight the danger in cases of obesity would appear to be the same in each. But there is an enormous difference between the two in one vital respect—the amount a person needs to consume of each before the appetite is appeased. A person may over-consume sugar very easily—but not apples.

Since Cleave began his pioneering work, other British doctors have also emphasized not only the dangers of processed sugars but also—and to a considerable extent this is the other side of the same coin—the benefits of dietary fiber. Fiber is that part of food derived from the cellular walls of plants such as sugar cane. In effect it is the skeleton of the plant, which is discarded in the refining process. Humans digest little of it, and until recently nutritionists and doctors therefore assumed that fiber had no value as food.

The identification of the value of dietary fiber has been principally a British achievement, a result, as Dr. Hugh Trowell has explained to me, of the British "having colonies where doctors could study the changing incidence of disease in time and in place and in various groups over a period of several years. History and geography favored us."

In the 1920s, Sir Robert McCarrison was Director of Research on Nutrition in India, then part of the British Empire. He was impressed by the superb health and physique of people in the state of Hunza in northernmost India, "whose sole food to this day consists of grains, vegetables, and fruits, with a certain amount of milk and butter, and meat only on feast days." Although they dwelt in primitive and harsh conditions, the Hunza in McCarrison's day were long-lived, and their illnesses were wholly unconnected with food. McCarrison contrasted this with the deplorable diet of Europeans fed on processed food. "Green vegetables are scanty, and such as there are, are often cooked to the point of almost complete extraction of their vitamin content and salts. White bread has largely replaced whole-wheat bread." He noted that a drop in infant and adult mortality accompanied the consumption of large quantities of whole cereals and potatoes in Belgium and Denmark during the First World War. Ironically, shortages forced the Danes to eat this healthy food; in peacetime cattle and swine ate the cereals and potatoes.

In his book *Nutrition and Health,* McCarrison also quoted studies by Dr. G. E. Friend, of special interest to me because Friend was the doctor—before my time—at my own school, one of those private schools the British call "public schools": Christ's Hospital. I well remember, in the 1950s, eating whole-wheat and "squashed fly" cookies (the latter named after the dried fruit they contained), the remnants of the doctor's campaign against refined food. Alas, the boys of my generation tended to flick this good food at each other, like miniature Frisbees. They were effective missiles. We preferred to eat sugary cookies from our private food lockers, having no idea of Dr. Friend's principles: "The deficiency of white bread in Vitamin B_1 is one of the most serious dietary deficiencies to which our populations are being subjected."

HEALTH IN BLACK AFRICA AND DURING WARS

Dr. Alec Walker, who left Great Britain for South Africa in 1938, has extended McCarrison's work. To discover the correlations between eating habits and disease patterns, Dr. Walker studied black Africans who moved from rural to urban areas and Indians moving from rural India to urban South Africa. He found that the move to urban areas reduced the life expectancy of middle-aged Africans and Indians. In 1974 he reported that the expectation of life of rural South

African blacks aged fifty exceeded that of whites of the same age. In rural India people of fifty usually died of infectious disease and had over 14 percent chance of reaching the age of seventy; in South Africa they usually died of coronary heart disease, strokes, cancer or diabetes and had only a 9 percent chance of reaching seventy. At an older age the differences are even more remarkable: "allowing for differences in population numbers, there are at least twenty times more Bantu over a hundred years old than whites."

Dr. Denis Burkitt, who worked for thirty years as a surgeon in East Africa, also observed that Africans living in rural areas did not get fat:

> In the 1920s doctors in East Africa reported that almost every African was slim. Even the soldiers who were liberally fed with traditional African food rarely appeared obese. In contrast urban Africans are commonly obese today and some of the overweight rulers are familiar figures on news media.

Like Dr. Burkitt, Dr. Walker became convinced that rural Africans and Indians who moved to urban areas began to suffer from obesity, and die from Western diseases, because their eating habits changed. Their traditional food, like the traditional food of virtually everybody in the world before the spread of industrialization in the West, was composed mainly of whole grain, rich not only in starches but also in protein, essential fats, fiber and other nutrients, lightly processed and lightly—if at all—cooked, together with vegetables and fruit. But in the urban areas they ate sugar and fat instead of cereal, and fewer vegetables. The dramatic difference was the virtual elimination of fiber.

Dr. Hugh Trowell was the first person to identify "Western diseases" as such. He worked in the same large teaching hospital in Uganda as Dr. Burkitt. His book *Noninfectious Diseases in Africa*, proposing that fiber gives protection against various diseases of the lower gut and bowel, was published in 1960; it sold twenty-seven copies in its first year. Undaunted, Trowell, with Burkitt, later identified seventeen diseases of previously uncertain origin that are common in the West and sent the list to thirty-four doctors working in teaching hospitals all over the world. Their response confirmed that these diseases, common among people with Western food habits, were rare among hunter-gatherers, and uncommon among peasants.

Dr. Cleave was independently accumulating his own evidence in favor of unprocessed cereal. In the Second World War, enemy attacks on Allied convoys reduced supplies of wheat to Great Britain from the United States. The government therefore stipulated that bread should contain much more of the whole wheat. The resulting brown "National Loaf" became the staple food from 1941 to 1955. In 1955, restrictions were lifted and the white loaf most people eat today was introduced. Cleave points out that between 1941 and 1954, mortality from diabetes fell by 54 percent, a finding similar to one made by Sir Robert McCarrison in the previous war.

The people of Singapore, faced with acute food shortages before the island fell to the Japanese in 1942, were compelled by the British authorities to eat whole brown rice, in order to save the 30 percent lost in the processing and polishing of rice. After one year of this regime infant mortality fell by half.

Cleave made two more remarkable discoveries in the Second World War. His brother, Surgeon-Captain Hugh Cleave, was a prisoner of war of the Japanese and the surgeon in charge of British prisoners in Hong Kong and later in Tokyo. British prisoners who worked on the Burma railway were fed whole brown rice and bran normally fed to swine. They did not suffer from ulcers of the stomach and gut. In Hong Kong, prisoners were fed processed white rice, and ulcers were common. The same prisoners were then transferred to Tokyo and fed brown rice; the ulcers vanished. Ulcers are often blamed on stress. But the ulcer-free prisoners of Tokyo were being held in a city that was largely destroyed by American bombing.

Cleave himself corresponded extensively with Germans taken prisoner on the Russian front. To the astonishment of German doctors in the front line, the closer their soldiers came to the Russians in the Stalingrad campaign, and the more anxiety, cold and fatigue they suffered, the fewer ulcers they had. The reason, Cleave came to realize, was that over-extended supply lines forced the soldiers to forage for food. They ate frozen raw vegetables, turnips in particular, and sour whole-meal bread. After returning to Germany, many of those who had ulcers before the Russian campaign suffered relapses.

More recently, in a study of 337 middle-aged men in London, Professor J.N. (Jerry) Morris of the London School of Hygiene and Tropical Medicine found that the men least subject to certain types of heart disease were those who ate most whole-wheat bread and breakfast cereal and most vegetable (as opposed to animal) fats, and whose energy intake from food was highest. The men most liable to heart attacks ate the least amount of cereal food.

For many years diabetics, rather like dieters, were told to avoid all carbohydrates. Now that it has been established that whole starchy food, with its fiber, is a protection against diseases caused by eating processed sugary food, diabetics are told to avoid only sugars, and to eat large quantities of whole starchy food. Whole foods can also improve the quality of the blood and so reduce the risk of heart attacks; they also prevent gallstones. Again, because of their bulk, whole foods are more satisfying than concentrated processed foods, and so they protect against obesity. Whether you are healthy, fit, fat, suffering from various Western diseases or at risk from them, or just want to gain a sense of well-being, the story is the same: eat whole food.

THE VALUE OF FIBER

Dietary fiber is that part of plants which is not digested by the small intestine. Fiber itself is essentially not a nutrient, but a package within which nutrients are contained. Foods that have fiber processed out of them lose nourishment with the fiber. This is one reason why whole foods including fiber are good for us, and processed foods, especially sugars, without fiber and with little or no nourishment, are bad for us.

Whole foods travel through the upper alimentary tract at a natural speed—relatively slowly. The fiber that binds the food allows its nutrients to be released into the bloodstream gradually, not in a rush. This is why starch (in the form of whole wheat bread, say) raises the blood sugar level, but at a natural speed; whereas sugar (in the form of candy or a soft drink, say) is liable to provoke an insulin response, with the eventual risk of obesity, diabetes or heart disease. Unlike processed sugar, the natural sugars in fruit are released slowly into the bloodstream. Dr. Kenneth Heaton has established that fruit juices, and even purées, can provoke an insulin response; the whole fruit is to be preferred.

The bulk of whole food gives the muscles of the intestines the work they are designed to do. The passage of fiber-rich food through the lower alimentary tract is comparatively faster. In the large bowel the fiber absorbs acids which, without the presence of fiber, become toxic and cause irritation and eventually the risk of cancer. With fiber, stools are soft, large, and easily evacuated. People who eat plenty of whole starchy fiber-rich food do not get constipated; fiber protects against piles, irritable bowels, and more serious conditions such as varicose veins, hernias, diverticular disease (rupture of the lower gut) and cancer of the large bowel, all caused by pressure, irritation or poisoning in the lower gut.

FIBER: HEALTHY, OR A SLIMMING AID?

Audrey Eyton's *The F-Plan Diet* has publicized fiber as a dieting aid. It is true that fiber-rich food can be more satisfying than processed food. For example, given the choice and asked to eat until they felt full, ten out of twelve people ate more white bread than whole-wheat bread. Including the energy value of the butter spread on the bread, those who ate the whole-wheat bread were on average satisfied with 665 calories; those who ate the white bread—with less fiber and a lot less nourishment in it—consumed 825 calories.

So there is something in what Mrs. Eyton says. The diet and exercise program developed by American nutritionist Nathan Pritikin is also healthier than most other popular diet regimes.

There is a danger, though, that dietary fiber will gain the status of a medicine. For example, after I wrote a feature for the *Sunday Times* about the value of fiber in whole food, the manufacturer of "Vita-Fibre" purchased a $15,000 advertisement extolling its fibrous quality. (I never learned how a pill can be fibrous; perhaps Vita-Fibre unfolds in the gut, like those little Japanese novelty items that, placed in water, swell into dragons.) Like vitamins and minerals, fiber is a natural part of whole food. It would be a disaster if it were generally perceived as a supplement to be sprinkled on top of processed food from which fiber—together with vitamins and minerals, and other nourishment—had been removed. Dr. Denis Burkitt put the point in a letter to me: "The right approach is a healthy diet, not a poor diet plus pills."

Another reason to stay away from fiber supplements, and to prefer whole food, is that dietary fiber is not one simple substance. Rather like the B complex of vitamins, dietary fiber is a whole series of substances, with different functions in the body. The pentoses, for example, are one part of fiber that increases the bulk of stools. People who eat bran or feed it to horses are aware of the effect of pentoses. Other components of fiber are lignin, pectin and gum. They have different properties. Pectin, for example, is good for the blood. A primary source of pentoses is cereal, and pectin is found in apples. The best policy is to eat a wide range of whole cereals, and fresh vegetables and fruit.

Unfortunately, most processed foods, even if higher-fiber, contain a lot of sugar. Heinz baked beans, for example, are high in fiber but also contain over 5 percent processed sugar. Beans baked at home are better for you. Kellogg's All-Bran contains over 15 percent processed sugar. For breakfast cereals, prefer shredded wheat, or sugar-free whole grain cereal eaten with plain yogurt and fruit.

It is a pity that Mrs. Eyton's recipes do not avoid processed food. Above all, the fault of the F-Plan is that her diets, of 1000 to 1500 calories, cannot contain enough nourishment. But anyone who eats whole-food versions of F-Plan recipes, eats around twice the amount of food stipulated, and at the same time takes plenty of the type of exercise recommended in the next chapter ("More Air! More Air!") will gradually and reliably lose fat and gain health.

THE VALUE OF CEREALS

The best food on earth is eaten by people who grow and eat their own food: peasants. In 1973 the Food and Agriculture Organization (FAO) and the World Health Organization (WHO) jointly published the results of a massive survey by Dr. J. Périssé of eating habits in eighty-five countries. This survey further documents the discoveries of Cleave, Burkitt, Trowell and other doctors, and reinforces our understanding of what makes food healthy.

The survey divided the eighty-five countries into four groups. The countries with least money, with 760 million inhabitants, had an average income per head per year of less than $100. The countries with most money, including the Western nations, had an income of $600 to $2600 per head per year. The two intermediate groups of countries, with 605 million inhabitants between them, had an average income of $100 to $600 per head per year.

The eating habits of the countries with least money proved to be profoundly different from those of the countries with most money. And the change from a "poor" or peasant pattern of eating to a "rich" or Western pattern proved to be systematic.

If food is categorized as protein, fat and carbohydrate—the conventional division—then the differences between the poor and the rich countries are remarkable enough. Measured as a percentage of total energy intake, protein consumption in the poor and rich countries was much the same: 11 to 12 percent. Fat consumption was massively different; 12 percent in the poor countries rising to over 40 percent in the rich countries (such as Great Britain and the United States). Carbohydrate consumption dropped correspondingly, from about 77 percent in the poor countries to 45 percent in the rich. This was confirmed by the McGovern report on dietary goals for the United States in 1977.

But these figures disguise the really massive difference in eating habits. Since the invention of agriculture about 10,000 years ago, whole cereals have been the staple food of mankind. All countries have developed a staple grain with which to make bread or its equivalent: wheat in Europe and North America, corn in the southern United States, rice in the East, and millet, rye, barley and oats elsewhere.

The cultivation of wheat from a hybrid of wild wheat and goat grass encouraged human settlement and, with it, the cultivation of other starchy foods: the pea and bean family (also known as pulses and legumes) and root vegetables (including tubers; notably, in recent times, the potato).

Naturally enough, therefore, the FAO survey showed that the poor nations obtain about 70 percent of their energy from the starch in whole carbohydrate foods: cereals and also peas, beans and root vegetables. These they eat lightly cooked or uncooked. Almost all the protein and fat they eat comes from these foods, as vegetable protein and vegetable fat. Only a tiny percentage of energy comes from animal protein and fats—about 7 percent in the poorest countries. The percentage of vegetable protein and fats amounts to about 16 percent. The remaining 7 percent is processed carbohydrate—mostly sugar, introduced recently. The main difference between these figures, researched in the early 1970s, and now, is that consumption of sugar is steadily rising.

In many countries most people do not get enough to eat. In the poorest countries many are starving, so they easily die from deficiency and infectious diseases. In other countries the land may be bad, the farming policies may be foolish or, as in any feudal society, the peasants may be subject to greedy rulers.

That said, a peasant in a settled society, whose wealth is his land and his produce, may neither need nor use much money. Though he may be classified as "poor" because he uses little money, in truth he may be well off. In good times and on good land, a peasant can enjoy plentiful, fresh whole cereals, vegetables and fruit, with meat and fish as occasional treats, and, in the matter of health rather than wealth, be rich.

The life expectancy of Greeks, at the age of forty, is notably higher than that of the British. On holiday in the Greek islands it is easy to know why. One day in 1983, for example, I visited Ioannis, who owns a farm in the mountains of Paros. He walks much of the day. He offers visitors a selection of what he grows: grapes, apples, cherries, walnuts, squash, peppers, eggplants. He shares his produce with the villagers a couple of miles below; he eats bread ground by the mill overlooking Naxos, drinks wine, eau de vie and cherry brandy made from his own fruit, and may buy meat, fish and cheese. To a Western European it may not be an exciting life; but it's a healthy life.

In the move from a peasant economy to industrialization, Western countries have come to depend upon processed food. Food is processed not for reasons of health, but for the imperatives of trade. The food that makes money for industry is food that keeps and travels well; and of all such foods sugars are the supreme commodity. Having no life, processed sugars do not rot.

At the same time, the rich countries grow prodigious quantities of grain. Michel Cépède, a French professor who works for the FAO, has calculated that whereas an inhabitant of the Third World eats somewhat over 400 pounds of cereal a year, North American and British people grow five times as much—nearly a ton of cereal a year—almost all of which is fed to animals raised for food. The amount of cereal actually eaten in North America, Great Britain and other Western countries is not much more than one-third of the amount in the Third World. Only rich countries can afford to breed animals for meat.

INDUSTRIALIZED PEOPLE EAT SUGARS AND FATS

The FAO figures show just how dramatically different Western food is from that of peasant countries. In the rich countries, industrialization has replaced cereals with processed foods, and with meat and dairy produce. Peasant countries affected by industrialization get the processed food without the meat and dairy produce. Ironically, it is the peasant countries too poor to eat much processed food that give us some guidance as to the food we need to keep our health. This table shows the contrast between the types of food eaten in peasant and in Western countries:

	Energy consumed (%)	
	Peasant	Western
Vegetable protein	7	4
Animal protein	4	8
Total	11	12
Vegetable fats	9	10
Animal fats	3	32
Total	12	42
Starches	70	28
Sugars	7	18
Total	77	46
Total vegetable foods	93	60
Total animal foods	7	40

OLD-FASHIONED GOOD SENSE ABOUT FOOD

The conventional chemistry of food divides it into protein, fat and carbohydrate, with energy value included. During this century, vitamins were identified and the value of vitamins and minerals established. So we are taught to think of foods as divided somewhat like a book, into a first part (energy—calories), a second part with three sections (protein, fat and carbohydrate) and then a lot of appendices with odd titles that tend to be skipped (vitamins, minerals). Unless we make a conscious decision not to do so, we are bound to think of food in this way, because engraved upon our brains is a lexicon in which calories are regarded with suspicion, protein is praised, carbohydrates are condemned (usually), fat is condemned (almost always), and vitamins are praised and touted (as a form of medicine); and, now, fiber is praised (also as a form of medicine—but where does it fit with the other categories?). No wonder we are often confused.

But there is a better way to classify food—the way it was done in Western countries before this century. Then food was divided into vegetable and animal food, whole and processed food, and fresh and stale food. We eat animal food for taste, and processed food for convenience, but we do not need them. Whole-wheat bread, legumes and root vegetables, well prepared and eaten fresh and lightly cooked, are rich in starch, true, but their classification as "carbohydrates" is arbitrary. Foods rich in starch are also rich in other nutrients. In different proportions, they also contain protein, essential fats, fiber, vitamins and minerals.

It is not necessary to be a vegetarian to be healthy. But it is necessary to rethink the relationship between animal and vegetable foods. "Meat and two veg" is the wrong balance. The chief ingredients in a meal should be cereal or vegetable: for example, the Italian staples of spaghetti and other pastas with olive oil, flavored in different combinations with vegetables or herbs or cheese or meat, is good food (and better still if the pasta is whole wheat). Meat and dairy produce, now a staple in the West, should merely accompany cereals and vegetables or should be eaten only occasionally. And while animal food eaten sparingly is of course nutritious, processed and stale food is always inferior to whole and fresh food.

All whole grains—wheat, corn, rice, millet, rye, oats—contain protein. So do the legumes—peas, beans, lentils. And so do tubers—potatoes, for example. Many dried beans have as high a protein content as meat; and nuts and seeds are rich in protein and also essential fats. We think of meat as protein and therefore as good for us, but much of the meat we eat could almost as well be classified as fat, rather than protein: more than half the calories in meat are from fat, with few exceptions. Even if it has no visible fat, the flesh of meat from animals that are reared in cages and get no exercise is shot through with fat; and animal fat, being highly saturated, is a cause of heart disease.

GOOD FOOD IS FOOD THAT GOES BAD

At the end of the chapter (pages 138–39) is a comparison taken from the standard textbook *The Composition of Foods* of the nutritive quality of five common foods commonly lumped together as "carbohydrates": potatoes (fresh, baked in their skins); a whole cereal (whole-wheat bread), compared with a processed cereal (white bread); a legume (lentils); and processed sugar.

First, look at the value of the much-despised potato. Potatoes are an important source of vitamin C, especially so when they are new and eaten with their skins. They are a useful source of magnesium and copper. Most importantly, they are a rich source of potassium. Many of us in the West consume too much sodium (in the form of salt) and not enough potassium. There is good evidence that excess sodium is a cause of high blood pressure, which in turn increases the risk of heart disease. There is new evidence, summarized in the last couple of years in *The Lancet*, that food rich in potassium can help to counteract the sinister effect of sodium. In this respect potatoes, together with most fresh vegetables and fruit, are a health-promoting food.

Whole-wheat bread is rich in no less than fourteen vitamins and minerals. By contrast, white bread has lost the vitamins occurring naturally in whole grain. Millers partially restore vitamins B_1 (thiamine), B_2 (riboflavin), and B_3 (niacin), together with iron and calcium, in order to enrich white flour, but it is still not as nourishing as whole wheat.

Like whole-wheat bread, and in common with many vegetables and fruits, lentils are an important source of a number of vitamins and minerals. And as a legume (one of the bean and pea family) lentils are also valuable as a source of protein—as are cereals.

In utter contrast to the whole foods in the table, processed sugar is empty of nourishment. Processing always drains nourishment from food; processed sugars are unique in having no nutritive value. We eat them at our peril.

The processing of food means that food can be preserved, and can travel and be stored for long periods of time. But processing is at the expense of nourishment. As a rule, good food is food that can go bad.

When nutrition experts say, as they so often do in newspapers and magazines, that we get all the nourishment we need from a "normal, balanced and varied" combination of foods, they are in one sense correct. But in a more important sense they are misleading. The fact is, that compared with the food eaten at any other time in history, the food we in the West have eaten for the last six generations is uniquely abnormal, unbalanced and artificially varied. The cuisine food based on meat, dairy produce, processed sugar and flour developed by the middle classes in Western Europe in the eighteenth century as one means of boasting of their riches is still considered good food in the United States, Great Britain, France and other Western countries. Cuisine food has caused the premature death of countless millions of people in the West. In the long view of history, cuisine food is the revenge of the black slaves on their masters, who gorged themselves on sugar and on the foods loaded with fat and sugar that they purchased with the profits of the slave trade. Nowadays, though, the Western diseases caused by eating processed sugars are, more and more, diseases of poor people in the West, for foods loaded with sugars, once a luxury, are now, together with foods loaded with animal fat, the most available, if not the cheapest, foods.

FRESH FOOD—AND FRESH AIR

The table "The Staff of Life" at the end of this chapter (pages 140–43) is a guide to peasant food—the healthy food that has been the staple food of people throughout history. Here are the general principles of healthy food.

Whole cereals, legumes and tubers are the natural staple foods of mankind. Of all these foods, whole-wheat bread is the single most valuable food that is produced in the West from a natural staple.

Vegetables and fruit, which contain starches or sugars and many vitamins and minerals, are a valuable complement to cereals, legumes and tubers, provided they are eaten whole and fresh, and raw or undercooked.

Vegetable protein and fat are always a better source of nourishment than animal protein and fats, which include dairy products. (Two exceptions are palm oil and coconut oil, which are highly saturated.) Nuts are a very valuable source of protein and fats, as are seeds.

Fresh food is always better than processed food. The closer food is to the earth the better. Vegetables are close to the earth; meat further away, meat from animals that eat meat, such as pigs, further away still.

The recommendations made by the McGovern committee in 1977 and the Royal College of Physicians in 1983 are all giant steps in the right direction. These reports follow the broad lines of a multitude of reports issued by expert committees of doctors and scientists since the 1960s, in America, Canada, Australia, New Zealand, various north European countries, and internationally representative bodies such as the World Health Organization. There is now general agreement that we in the West should eat less fats and a lot less sugars and salt; that we should prefer protein and fats from vegetable sources; and that we should eat plenty of whole, fresh cereal produce, vegetables and fruit. We eat about the right amount of protein, but we should get more of it from vegetable sources.

But how much less, and how much more? The expert committees have all tried to work out recommendations which could be achieved by entire populations, with the cooperation of government and industry. That is to say, their recommendations are honorable compromises, since many of the committees have had to deal with pressure from government and industry, which want to maintain the status quo, or only marginally modify our current Western eating habits.

Peasant communities get most of their protein and fats from the cereal staples that they eat, together with small amounts of lean meat. We in Western countries are bound to eat more fats; even the Japanese, renowned for their low-fat diet, are eating more fat nowadays. Besides, the fats in whole foods are nourishing. So it is not sensible to recommend that we eat only 12 percent of our calories in the form of fat. An ideal is about twice that amount, or 25 percent, provided that most fats eaten are of vegetable origin (and therefore contain a lot of polyunsaturates, including essential fats).

So the goal is to eat rather less fats than recommended by the expert committees and, at the same time, to eat rather more whole carbohydrate. It is practically impossible to eat too much cereal, or vegetables, or fruit in whole form: all are filling.

Again, peasant communities cannot be an exact guide to the amount of processed carbohydrate we should eat. But, there again, my own view is that recommendations to cut intake of processed sugars by half can be misleading, because this can suggest that halving our present intake is an ideal, which it is not. The ideal is to eat no processed sugars at all: zero. Nor is it sensible to reserve cakes, cookies, and chocolate, say, for the occasional treat: the best policy is to get over the habit of eating sugars, which takes about a month or so, after which food with processed sugar added tastes sickly. Likewise with salt; the best policy is to stop using it in cooking, stop adding it to food, and so become accustomed to the natural taste of food. The salts naturally present in whole food supply all our needs—potassium as well as sodium. So any figure for "processed carbohydrate" in a list of goals is not an ideal, but merely allows for the fact that it is not really possible completely to avoid it.

GOALS FOR HEALTHY FOOD

Here are the goals I propose, given the conventional division of foods into protein, fat and carbohydrate, but also making the vital distinction between foods of animal origin (including

	Peasant (%)	Western (%)	McG/RCP[1] (%)	Goal (%)
Vegetable protein	7	4	—	7
Animal protein[2]	4	8	—	5
Total	11	12	12	12
Vegetable fats	9	10	—	15
Animal fats	3	32	—	10
Total	12	42	30	25
Starches, etc.[3]	70	28	48	55
Sugars[4]	7	18	10	8
Total	77	46	58	63
Total vegetable foods	93	60	75	85
Total animal foods	7	40	25	15

1. No separate figures given for vegetable and animal.
2. Including dairy produce.
3. Starches mainly; also sugars from fruit, etc.
4. Processed sugars.

dairy produce) and foods of vegetable origin. Also given are
the current figures for peasant countries, for Western countries, and those recommended by expert committees like the
McGovern and the Royal College of Physicians committees
(indicated as McG/RCP).

In the Harveian Oration given to the Royal College of
Physicians in London, in October 1982, Sir Richard Doll,
having linked obesity, diabetes and high risk of heart attacks
as diet-related diseases, had this to say:

> Whether the object is to avoid cancer, coronary
> heart disease, hypertension, diabetes, diverticular
> disease, duodenal ulcer, or constipation, there is
> broad agreement among research workers that the
> type of diet that is least likely to cause disease is
> one that provides a high proportion of calories in
> whole-grain cereals, vegetables, and fruit; provides
> most of its animal protein in fish and poultry; limits
> the intake of fats, and, if oils are to be used, gives
> preference to liquid vegetable oils; includes very
> few dairy products, eggs, and little refined sugar.

In 1984 I asked Sir Richard if he would say anything differently. "I would strengthen that statement now," he told
me. "The evidence now is even stronger than it was two years
ago."

Some cookbooks have now been written designed to
encourage us to enjoy delicious food which is also healthy.
Meanwhile, a couple of tips from Dr. Denis Burkitt go a long
way to help. After recommending breakfasts of whole-wheat
bread or sugar-free cereal, he goes on to say:

> If I were asked to make one change only in Western
> diets it would be that we should eat three times as
> much bread but almost never white. The changes to
> make in the main meal would be to eat four or five
> times as much potato and vegetable as meat, and
> the potatoes should not be peeled, and not cooked
> or eaten in fat.

Representatives of the food industry who want to see no real change in our eating habits claim that we need lots of fats, sugars and salt to make our food "palatable." Nonsense. Processing foods masks the true, delicious taste of whole food. I've never met anybody who switched to wholewheat bread and then switched back to white bread.

The most obvious sign that our food, in the West, has been drained of nourishment is the obesity all around. The worse the food, the fatter people get, as they try to get enough nourishment. The prevalence of obesity, diabetes and heart disease tells us it is time for a change—to good food and plenty of it.

In the first chapter of this book ("Confessions of a Dieter") I quoted a befuddled passage from one of Dr. Robert Atkins' diet books in which he says that if all else fails, a trip to the Mediterranean is recommended. It "always seems to help with weight reduction. It may be something in the soil." And I mentioned my month's holiday in Greece, during which I lost 8 pounds. Well, there is no cuisine food in Greece. Greek food remains peasant food, and authentic Greek food is the healthiest in Europe. During my long stay I got as close to the guidelines to healthy food outlined above as I ever had in my life. Dr. Atkins' shot in the dark in fact hits the target.

What I also enjoyed in Greece that summer was plenty of fresh air. And for everybody who wants to lose fat while eating plenty of good food, the recipe is: peasant food, and more air.

THE STAFF OF LIFE

Throughout history, people all over the world have relied on whole fresh foods of vegetable origin as their staples, with foods of animal origin usually playing the minor role. The idea that our primeval ancestors dined off mastodon and saber-toothed tiger every day is a myth: examination of fossil teeth shows that early man and woman spent more time gathering than hunting.

Since the beginnings of agriculture 10,000 years ago, people have cultivated vegetables, pulses, fruit and cereals and have made some form of bread the chief staple food, while also consuming meat, fish, milk and other dairy produce, usually sparingly. As societies became richer and more sophisticated in the West, during the past 300 years or so, the consumption of foods of animal origin tended to increase among the better-off. But hunter-gatherers, pastoralists and peasants alike, generally relied mainly on foods of vegetable origin.

The Industrial Revolution, with all its consequences, has created a unique and catastrophic aberration in the eating habits of people in Western countries, during the last 100–150 years. During this century the consumption of bread, cereals, vegetables and fish has dropped, while the consumption of sugars, fats, meat and highly processed foods of all kinds has risen. These foods, drained of nourishment and eventually toxic in their effect, eaten in the quantities they are now eaten in Western countries, are the main single cause of the Western diseases we mostly suffer and die from.

The good news is that we do not need to become peasants in order to eat well. We can take advantage of the modern benefit of fast transport, together with the relatively harmless methods of preserving food (freezing and drying), and enjoy the most varied, most delicious and also most nourishing food ever available. A healthy way of eating means less profits for the food industry, but it is also likely to mean more money in your pocket: generally speaking, animal and processed foods are more expensive than vegetable and fresh foods, even though some individual healthy foods cost more than the mass-produced inferior item.

This table lists fifty nourishing foods that will give health and prevent disease, and that are, together with regular vigorous exercise, proof against obesity.

The first section is of bread and cereals, including some ready-to-eat breakfast cereals. Of all these, whole-meal bread is the most valuable of all: it is rich in many vitamins and minerals, as well as protein, fiber, and essential fats (EFAs). The most nourishing breakfast cereal you can make yourself from a mixture of whole grains, dried fruit, nuts, seeds and fresh fruit; in Europe this is called muesli.

Most vegetables—root and green vegetables, salads and pulses—are nourishing; the list gives only fifteen representative examples. A raw vegetable or fruit contains the most nourishment. Always prefer the whole, fresh item: for example, a new potato eaten with its skin contains much more vitamin C and fiber. The secret with cooking is a gentle touch. Steaming is best. Vitamins are lost with boiling, but undercooked vegetables that remain crisp retain much of their original nourishment. In salads, don't be afraid of the avocado: it is exceptionally rich in vitamins and minerals, and its fats are low in saturated fatty acids (SFAs).

It's worth noting that all fifty items in the following lists are good sources of potassium (the mineral whose initial is K). People in Western countries not only consume far too much sodium (Na) but also not enough potassium, and so the natural balance between these two minerals is destroyed. Avoid canned vegetables and fruit, and at all costs avoid canned or packet soups when these are heavy in salt, as all but brands marked "low salt" are.

Like vegetables, most fruits are good news. Dried fruits are of course high in calories.

The problem with dairy produce is saturated fats. The movement to low-fat products and to skimmed milk is healthy. Eat butter and cheese sparingly.

Nuts and seeds of all types are very nourishing, and the three examples are fairly representative of many others. The fats in nuts and seeds are nourishing (EFAs); and these natural foods are very good sources of folic acid (Fo) and of iron (Fe) and zinc (Zn), three nutrients people in Western countries are generally short of.

Vegetarians tend to be healthier than people who eat meat and meat products. But some food of animal origin is exceptionally nutritious. The way to avoid getting fat is to get fit. Likewise, the way to avoid unhealthy fat in food of animal origin is to eat fit flesh. This means fish, game animals and game birds, above all. Not only is the flesh of animals, fish and birds that live free lower in fat, but its fats are high in life-giving essential fatty acids (EFAs). Fatty fish are exceptionally nutritious. Eat only free-range poultry, and trim its fat and skin off.

The closer a food is to its natural environment of earth,

TABLE 2: THE NOURISHMENT IN FIVE FOODS

Figures are for 100 grams, which is 3½ ounces (equivalent to a medium-size potato, or three thin slices of bread). Due to methods of analysis and micronutrient content, the percentages of nutrients do not always add up to 100. Figures in bold type: nutrients of which the food is a good source.[1]

		Potatoes, baked	Bread, whole-meal	Bread, white, enriched	Lentils, boiled	Sugar, processed
Water	%	73.0	36.4	35.8	72.0	tr
Protein	%	2.6	**10.5**	**8.7**	**7.8**	tr
Fat	%	0.1	3.0	3.2	tr	0
Starches	%	**21.0**	**39.7**	**45.9**	**16.2**	0
Sugars	%	0.6	2.0	2.0	0.8	**100** [2]
Fiber	%	**2.5**	**8.0**	**2.7**	**3.7**	0
Energy	cals	95	243	255	100	394
VITAMINS:						
A (Carotene)	mcg	tr	tr	tr	20.0	0
Thiamine (B$_1$)	mg	**0.1**	**0.25**	**0.25** [3]	0.07	0
Riboflavin (B$_2$)	mg	0.04	**0.12**	**0.12** [3]	0.06	0
Niacin (B$_3$)	mg	**1.2**	**2.8**	**2.3** [3]	0.6	0
Pyridoxine (B$_6$)	mg	**0.18**	**0.14**	0.04	0.11	0
Cobalamin (B$_{12}$)	mcg	0	0	0	0	0
Folic Acid (B)	mcg	10	**22.0**	**6.0**	1.0	0
Pantothenic acid (B)	mg	0.2	**0.6**	0.3	0.3	0
Biotin (B)	mcg	tr	**6.0**	**1.0**	0	0

C (Ascorbic acid)	mg	15 [4]	tr	tr	tr	0
D	mcg	0	0	0	0	0
E	mg	0.1	0.2	tr	0	0
MINERALS:						
Sodium (Na)	mg	8.0	540 [2]	540 [2]	tr	0
Potassium (K)	mg	680	273	100	250	2.0
Calcium (Ca)	mg	9.0	100	100	25.0	2.0
Magnesium (Mg)	mg	29.0	93.0	26.0	25.0	tr
Phosphorus (P)	mg	48.0	220	97.0	120	tr
Iron (Fe)	mg	0.8	2.3	1.7 [3]	2.1	tr
Copper (Cu)	mg	0.18	0.3	0.1	0.2	tr
Zinc (Zn)	mg	0.3	2.0	0.8	1.0	0

1. Good source: 7–8 percent or more of U.S. RDA or similar recommendation.
2. Not valuable at this level. We consume too much sugar, and sodium (as salt).
3. Only enriched bread (with these nutrients added back) is a good source.
4. Vitamin C content of vegetables and fruit varies: fresh, lightly cooked have highest values.

Chief sources of information: *McCance and Widdowson's The Composition of Foods*, edited by A. A. Paul and D. A. T. Southgate (HMSO, 1978); *Composition of Foods* (Agriculture Handbook No. 8, USDA, 1975); *Recommended Dietary Allowances* (9th edition, National Academy of Sciences, 1980).

TABLE 3: THE STAFF OF LIFE—

Note: Due to methods of analysis and micronutrient content,

	Water	Protein	Fats	Starches	Sugars	Fiber	Energy
BREAD, CEREALS	(%)	(%)	(%)	(%)	(%)	(%)	(cals[1])
Bread (whole-meal)	36	10	3	40	2	8	243
Cheerios	5	15	6	65	3	5	391
Flour (whole-meal)	14	13	2	63	2	6	318
Granola	3	12	27	40	15 [2]	7	480
Pasta (whole-meal, cooked)[3]	70	3	1	21	tr	2	111
Puffed rice	3	6	1	90	tr	2	402
Puffed wheat	2	14	1	67	2	15	325
Rice (brown, cooked)[3]	70	2	1	25	tr	1	119
Shredded wheat	7	10	3	67	1	12	324
Wheatgerm	6	30	8	33	8	15	350
VEGETABLES, SALADS, PULSES							
Avocados	68	4	23	tr	2	2	223
Beans (butter) (boiled)[4]	70	7	tr	18	tr	5	95
Beans (lima, kidney, mung)[5]	70	8	1	19	tr	2	111
Broccoli	90	3	tr	tr	2	4	18
Brussels sprouts	91	3	tr	tr	2	3	18
Cabbage	93	2	tr	tr	2	3	15
Corn (sweet)	74	3	1	16	2	4	91
Lentils	72	8	tr	16	1	4	100
Peppers (sweet) (raw)	95	1	tr	tr	2	1	14
Potatoes	78	1	tr	19	tr	1	80
Potatoes (& skins) (baked)	73	2	tr	21	1	3	95
Spinach	86	5	1	tr	1	6	30
Squash, zucchini	96	tr	tr	tr	2	2	8
Sweet potatoes	72	2	1	13	9	3	105
Tomatoes (raw)	93	1	tr	tr	3	2	14
FRUIT							
Apples[6]	84	tr	tr	tr	12	3	45
Apricots[6]	89	1	tr	0	7	2	31
Bananas	75	1	tr	3	16	4	79
Dates (dried)	22	2	1	0	66	9	275
Figs	85	1	tr	0	10	3	41
Grapes	81	1	tr	0	16	1	65
Melons[7]	93	1	tr	0	5	1	21
Oranges	87	1	tr	0	9	2	36
Plums	86	1	tr	0	10	2	40
Raisins	22	2	tr	0	68	7	280

FIFTY COMMON NUTRITIOUS FOODS

percentages do not always add up to 100.

Vitamins	Minerals	Pluses	Minuses
Good sources of	Good sources of		
B1 B2 B3 B6 Fo Pa Bi	K Ca Mg P Fe Cu Zn	EFAs	Salt
B1 B2 B3 B6 Fo Pa	K Ca Mg P Fe Cu Zn		
B1 B2 B3 B6 Fo Pa Bi E	K Ca Mg P Fe Cu Zn	EFAs	
B1 B2 B3 B6 Fo Pa	K Mg P Fe Cu Zn	EFAs	Sugars
B1 B2 B3 B6 Fo Pa Bi	K Mg P Fe Cu Zn		Salt (if added)
B1 B2 B3	K P Cu		
B3 E	K Mg P Fe Cu Zn		
B1 B2 B3 B6 Bi	K Ca Mg K	EFAs	Salt (if added)
B1 B3 B6 Fo	K Mg P Fe Cu Zn		
B1 B2 B3 B6 Fo Pa Bi E	K Mg P Fe Cu Zn	EFAs	
A B1 B2 B3 B6 Fo Pa Bi C E	K Mg Cu	Low SFAs	
Fo	K Mg Cu Zn		
B1 Fo	K Mg Fe		
A B1 B6 Fo C E	K Ca Fe		
A B6 Fo C E	K		
A B6 Fo C	K Ca Mg		
	K Mg Fe Zn		
	K Mg P Fe Cu		
A C E	K		
B1 B3 B6 C	K Mg Cu		
B1 B3 B6 C	K Mg Cu		
A B2 B6 Fo C E	K Ca Mg Fe		
A Fo	K		
A Fo C E	K		
A B1 C E	K		
C	K		
A	K		
A B6 Fo	K Mg		
B3 B6 Pa	K Mg Fe		
B6	K		
	K		
A Fo C	K		
Fo C	K		
A	K		
B1 B6 E	K Ca Mg P Fe Cu		

TABLE 3 *(continued)*

	Water	Protein	Fats	Starches	Sugars	Fiber	Energy
DAIRY PRODUCE							
Milk (cows) (skimmed)	91	3	tr	0	5	0	33
Yogurt (plain) (low-fat)	89	4	1	0	6	0	41
NUTS, SEEDS							
Almonds[8]	6	19	55	0	4	14	590
Peanuts	6	26	49	5	3	8	570
Sesame seeds	6	19	50	13	5	8	590
MEAT, FISH, POULTRY							
Chicken (roast)[9]	68	25	6	0	0	0	148
Cod (baked)	79	19	1	0	0	0	101
Herring (grilled)	66	20	12	0	0	0	199
Mackerel (baked)	64	20	15	0	0	0	223
Oyster (raw)	87	11	1	tr	0	0	51
Rabbit (stewed)	64	27	8	0	0	0	179
Salmon (poached)	66	20	13	0	0	0	197
Tuna (in water)	70	28	1	0	0	0	127
Turkey (roast)[10]	68	29	3	0	0	0	140
Venison (roast)	57	35	7	0	0	0	198

Notes
1. Calories are for 100 grams (3½ ounces).
2. Sugars content varies according to recipe.
3. If white, lower vitamin and mineral values.
4. Cooking method always boiled unless stated.
5. Values apply to other beans (white, red, etc.).
6. Values for raw fruit with peel when eatable, but without core or stones, unless stated.
7. Not watermelons, which have lower values.
8. Fresh, kernels only, unsalted.
9. Meat only; all skin and fat trimmed off.

Vitamins	Minerals	Pluses	Minuses
B2 Bi	K Ca P		
B2	K Ca P		
B1 B2 B3 Fo E	K Ca Mg P Fe Zn	EFAs	Energy dense
B1 B2 B3 Fo Pa E	K Mg P Fe Zn	EFAs	Energy dense
B3 Fo	K Fe Zn	EFAs	Energy dense
B2 B3 Pa	K Fe Zn		
B3 B6 B12 Bi	K Mg P		
B1 B2 B3 B6 B12 Fo Pa Bi D	K Mg P Fe	EFAs	
A B1 B2 B3 B6 B12 Fo Pa Bi D	K Mg P Cu	EFAs	
A B1 B2 B3 B12 Bi	K Ca Mg P Fe Cu Zn		
B2 B3 B6 B12 Pa	P Fe		
A B1 B2 B3 B6 B12 Fo Pa Bi D	K P	EFAs	
B2 B3 B6 B12 Fo Pa D E	K P		
B2 B3 B6 B12 Pa Bi	K Mg P Fe Zn		
B1	K Mg P Fe	EFAs	

Key:
Vitamins A: Carotene. B1: Thiamine. B2: Riboflavin. B3: Niacin. B6: Pyridoxine. B12: Cyanocobalamin. Fo: Folic acid. Pa: Pantothenic acid. Bi: Biotin. C: Ascorbic Acid. D and E usually known only by letters.
Minerals K: Potassium. Ca: Calcium. Mg: Magnesium. P: Phosphorus. Fe: Iron. Cu: Copper. Zn: Zinc

Chief sources of information: *McCance and Widdowson's The Composition of Foods*, edited by A. A. Paul and D. A. T. Southgate (HMSO, 1978); *Composition of Foods* (Agriculture Handbook No. 8, USDA, 1975) *Recommended Dietary Allowances* (9th edition, National Academy of Sciences, 1980).

or water or air, the more nourishing it will be. The more highly processed a food is, the less nourishing it will be. Nowadays it is hard to find perfect foods: almost all the food we eat has been touched by pesticides or chemicals of some kind. But short of growing and breeding your own, the following lists give a guide to some of the common foods that can provide us with the staff of life.

5

More Air! More Air!

Nothing affects cheerfulness less than wealth and nothing more than health. Let us seek to maintain cheerfulness. Without appropriate daily exercise no one can remain healthy, because satisfactory completion of all living functions requires movements of the parts concerned as well as of the whole. Aristotle was right to say "life is motion."

—Arthur Schopenhauer
Aphorisms on the Wisdom of Life

The narrower and more limited our lives become, the more vitally necessary people will find it to satisfy their longing for freedom in the hazard of their athletic performance.

—Roger Bannister
The First Four Minutes

OXYGEN: THE VITAL FUEL

Wealth, power and fame have their rewards, but most people who live well manage without them. Sooner or later we all find out that the most valuable prize in life is not a rare external object but a common blessing most of us are born with: our health.

We in the West have had a negative attitude toward health. We spend the first part of our lives thinking nothing of it, and the second part afraid of losing it. We have been preoccupied not with good health but with ill health; not with well-being but with disease. An unorthodox but apt definition of "technology" is "a means whereby we avoid experiencing our own lives." Medical technology—the medicine of drugs and surgery where the money, power, newspaper headlines and Nobel Prizes are—discourages us from being responsible for our own health. Our attitude toward doctors and surgeons is like that of the little child who cries out, "Mummy, take the pain away!" We tend to think of disease as a visitation, as bad luck, as something for which we have no responsibility.

We generally associate the concept of disease with what is in fact only one type of disease: infections, which indeed can be checked or cured by modern medicine. But we ignore deficiency diseases, caused by lack of nourishment from food, because we assume they do not exist in the West. And we fear the "degenerative" diseases of the heart, lungs and blood vessels, and of the gut. In some way we imagine that these, too, are visitations, whereas they are principally caused by the circumstances in which we live and by our own habits.

It was not always so. The awareness that our good health is our responsibility, a treasure to be protected, is contained in our language. The words "salute" and "salutation" derive from *salus,* the Latin word for "health." It also means "safety." The common French and Italian greetings— *"Salut!"* and *"Salute!"*—are wishes for good health and well-being. In America and Britain, greetings are more neutral. But on formal occasions, speakers will propose each other's health; and sometimes over drinks, if the occasion seems right, you may toast a friend with the words "your good health." The old knowledge is still there, although half-buried.

As with good health, so with the universal element in our environment: air. People who spend most of their time sitting or lying down, especially town and city dwellers, pay no attention to air. After all, as well as being everywhere, it is invisible. The irony is that without air we die within five minutes, but only in extremity do we remember its value. On the point of drowning, the swimmer has one thought in mind; likewise, the person hemmed in by street crowds. The cry is the same. "More air! More air!"

Oxygen is that part of air which is vital to all the functions of the body. Just as fuel is burned by combining with the oxygen in the air, to provide energy in the form of heat, so oxygen transforms the fuel we eat—food—into all the types of energy that make up life itself—not, of course, in a flame, but by agents in the body that oxidize the food. The dictionary defines "food" as "what one takes into the system to maintain life and growth." This is why the great nutritionist Sir Robert McCarrison wrote: "Strictly speaking oxygen and water are to be regarded as foods, for of all the supplies on which the cells of the body are dependent they are the chief."

Which comes first, then: food or oxygen? In one sense the question has no meaning, for we need both, just as a domestic fire cannot exist without both fuel and oxygen. And just as a domestic fire may burn well and brightly with different amounts of fuel and with different drafts, so we can live and thrive at very different levels of energy balance, between the energy supplied by food and that of oxygen.

THE DESIRE TO BE FIT

In a vital sense, though, oxygen comes first. The purpose of the newborn infant's first cry is to take air into its lungs. Most people in Western countries are in a double bind. Not only do they suffer from eating highly processed, unnatural foods, they also suffer because they do not take the exercise that was a natural part of life before the car was invented. To free oneself from this bind, the first step is to take in more oxygen by means of appropriate exercise. The most important thing about food is not quantity, but quality. But with oxygen, quantity counts; almost all of us will thrive if we get more of it. And once we start to use more oxygen, remarkable things begin to happen.

In spring 1982 I launched what became known as the Fun Runner '82 project with *Running* magazine, in London. Having started to jog in 1978, and run my first marathon in Paris in 1980, I began to write a column for *Running*. In 1981 I launched the London 1982/50 project. The title was meant to convey the project's aim: to train fifty men and women for the second London marathon in 1982. The project worked; and so I and about a dozen of the 1982/50 participants decided to encourage a group of absolute beginners to train, not for a marathon, but to complete the *Sunday Times* National Fun Run five months later, in September. This was Fun Runner '82.

We reckoned that the Hyde Park Fun Run, which is two and a half miles long, was an attainable goal. "To qualify, you have to be an absolute beginner," I wrote.

> I'm looking for people who have never kept fit on any regular basis. I shall be especially interested if you're overweight, or smoke, or have had any history of debilitating illness, or in general feel that you're in such bad shape that the Fun Run seems an Everest.

The applications poured in, from couples, from men, from women.

> We suddenly realized we were getting old and out of condition when we got a dog that needed a lot of exercise.

This was from a couple aged twenty-eight. An ex-smoker who was toying with the idea of becoming an ex-drinker wrote:

> After the excesses of Christmas I looked into the mirror and was horrified to see a flabby 5'11", 196 pound, balding local government officer. Two of these factors could not be reversed, but I decided to do something about my weight and fitness.

Most of the letters were from people who thought, correctly, that they were overweight. One mother said that her family loved swimming, but that she no longer went because she was ashamed of her size. Two other letters from women said:

> I am twenty-eight, and have progressively got less and less fit during the last five years. My energy output is very low as I have an office job that entails sitting down all day. The time has come when I would love to be fit again.

And (from a middle-aged mother):

> Is this the answer to the feeling that my waist is sinking into my hips, is this the self-discipline I have vaguely been feeling I need?

Most of the overweight people were women whose weight had increased to 140 pounds or more, and who had discovered that dieting doesn't work. Some had been humiliated by the emphasis on competitive sport at school:

> I was overweight during my school years and pretty useless at sports, always being the one that the coach had to wait for after the cross-country.

Many wrote of lost energy. These letters were wistful, moving, sometimes resigned, a few despairing.

Eventually I received 130 applications. The first 84 were analyzed; four were from asthma sufferers, three from people with diagnosed high blood pressure. One person had a heart murmur. Other conditions included a pulmonary embolism (recovered), slipped disks (two), back problems, bronchitis, hernia, curvature of the spine and epilepsy. One of the most touching letters said:

> Medically the last eighteen months have been rotten. Head, leg and shoulder injuries and an unknown virus took it out of me spiritually as well as physically. However, I feel much better now, except that I feel the strain of being very overweight.

Of the eighty-four, twenty-two smoked; twenty-three had

given up; forty-nine were definitely overweight; thirty-eight had taken no exercise since school; and forty said they had exercised "a bit." Their ages ranged from eighteen to fifty-five; most people were in their thirties and forties. The average age was early to middle thirties.

HOW TO SAVE YOUR OWN LIFE

Eventually sixty-four people were chosen to take part in Fun Runner '82. The fittest participant was, at fifty-five, the oldest: John Routledge, a company director. The previous summer he had been given an executive checkup. He was a bit alarmed at his blood pressure, but was told that it was not unusual for his age. Then a couple of months later he had a massive heart attack and clinically "died." Afterward, in hospital, he remembered a conversation with a friend playing snooker; he had leaned over the table to play a ball and couldn't reach. "Your undercarriage is in the way, John," said his friend. Out of the hospital, John started to jog, and eat fresh food. He had lost about 30 pounds and was doing five-mile runs when I met him. His experience as a runner should have disqualified him from joining the project, but his experience of heart disease and his subsequent decision to save his own life would, I thought, be valuable. Vic Burrowes, one of the applicants, had written:

> If I am selected for your programme it could change my whole way of life. You said it might seem an Everest to some people. At the moment I would liken it to climbing the whole Himalayan range.

I was interested to see what would happen to Vic.

TESTING FITNESS

The participants in the project all agreed to undertake a series of tests during the five-month training program. The physiological tests, based on the work of Professor Per-

Olof Åstrand in Stockholm, were supervised by Ted Charlesworth and Kevin Sykes of the Human Performance Laboratory at Chester College and had already been used to test the fitness of the Cheshire fire service and police. They were carried out three times: at the start of the project, at the midpoint and at the end of the twenty-one weeks.

As well as taking measurements of height, weight and various parts of the body, we tested blood pressure; body fat percentage (nonessential fat); lung capacity; heart rate; cardiorespiratory fitness (fitness of the heart and lungs); and, finally, "fitness category." Everybody wanted to know "How fit am I?" Fitness category was determined by measuring the fitness of the heart and lungs in terms of the body's capacity to use oxygen, and resulted in the following grades: "excellent," "good," "average," "below average," and—rock bottom—"poor." This grading was based on measurements of tens of thousands of people carried out in Dallas, Texas, by Dr. Kenneth Cooper, founder of the Aerobics Institute.

I was also interested to know how far individuals' moods, attitudes and personality might change as a result of exercise and increasing fitness. So Dr. Barrie Gunter, a research psychologist with special knowledge of sport, asked everyone to fill in a long questionnaire at the beginning and end of the project. This was the "Cattell 16 Personality Factor" test, a standard method of measuring shifts in personality.

I myself devised a questionnaire for everyone to fill in at the midpoint of the project. This was designed to find out why people had joined Fun Runner '82, what they were getting out of it, and whether their eating and sleeping habits were changing. I also wanted to find out if people's moods changed as a result of exercise.

THE COST OF HEART DISEASE

The physiological tests are usually called "fitness tests." I prefer the name "health tests," for what they measure is the health and strength of the heart, lungs and blood vessels. They do not check the health of the whole body, but nonetheless they are important.

It seems to me that these tests, which take about twenty-five minutes to carry out and are suitable for all able-bodied people whatever their level of fitness, should be available as part of a physician's routine examination and in public health clinics in schools and the community.

Around a million people die every year in America from heart disease, stroke and associated diseases. The figure in Britain is around 250,000 a year. It is interesting that Americans are moving toward a healthy diet and are taking more exercise, and in the last fifteen years the rate of deaths from heart disease in America has dropped by over 25 percent, while in Britain the rate of death from heart disease has not changed significantly in the last twenty years.

Leading heart disease specialists such as Professor Jeremiah Stamler, Professor Barry Lewis, and Professor Geoffrey Rose believe that healthy food, exercise and non-smoking would prevent between 30 and 90 percent of deaths from heart disease. We still live in a world, though, where prevention, though cheaper than treatment, is less glamorous, even when the immensely expensive treatment involving coronary bypass, heart transplants or plastic hearts is unlikely to be effective. To give just one American statistic, Professor Jeremiah Stamler tells me that in 1983, 180,000 bypass operations were performed at an average cost of $35,000 each—a total of $630 million.

The initial series of physiological tests showed that on average the Fun Runners were a bit overweight and overfat; that their blood pressure was noticeably above the "ideal" of 120/80 for women (at 127/91) and somewhat higher for men (at 137/93); and that fitness level was about "average" for men and a bit "below average" for women. "Average" fitness is nothing to be satisfied about; it is what it says, the average for a basically sedentary population. The averages concealed a wide range of fitness. Of the twenty-five men assessed before they started to exercise, six were "below average" and two "poor." The women's fitness level was lower; of the thirty-two women measured, five were "below-average" and ten "poor." The "poor" rating means you are liable to get out of breath running a bath.

The Fun Runners were formed into six teams, of ten to a dozen people each. Experience shows that this is a good number for a team and allows for a few people to be absent without spoiling the group. Each team had two trainers. These were mostly people from the now-completed London 1982/50 project who had told me that they had gained so much from their nine months that they wanted to put some of their enthusiasm, time and experience into inspiring others.

Once a week every team met with their trainers. Once a month everybody came together on a Saturday morning in Hyde Park for a "family" run. Special T-shirts were printed. Everybody was asked to exercise four times a week, preferably evenly spaced, and to keep a diary in which he or she recorded the times and distances that were covered.

SLOW AND STEADY

When starting an exercise program, it is crucial to take it easy at first and build up slowly. At first all the participants were asked to jog and walk just over a mile, stopping whenever they liked. (Unfit people can usually run 200 to 400 yards without stopping.) As time went on, they were encouraged to jog, and then run, further and faster, but always in their own time and at their own speed. The secret in this kind of training is to take your pulse rate and check to see that it is neither too high nor too low. (A guide to a training program that able-bodied people can use is the table "Health Through Fitness," on pages 189–91.)

At the midpoint of the project everybody was given the second fitness test. Allan Appleton, a forty-six-year-old company director, who had started the project with "below average" fitness, had risen to "excellent." In five months he was to lose 22 pounds in weight and 30 percent of his nonessential body fat. But for him the main benefits at the halfway stage were:

> Many, and much appreciated: a tremendous increase in fitness and well-being, the previously unknown pleasure of running with members of my family. I will, for the rest of my life, run and exercise regularly.

You don't often hear this kind of enthusiasm about a diet. Allan's loss of weight and nonessential fat was unusually high.

I spent most time during the project with the "Inner" team in central London, which included John Routledge and Vic Burrowes. At the halfway stage, after eleven weeks, their results were:

	Age	Body Weight (lbs.)		Nonessential Body Fat (%)		Fitness Category	
		Before	after	Before	after	Before	after
Cinnia Bermingham	36	127	121	16	14	5	2
Victor Burrowes	46	178	155	18	14	3	2
Tim Burton	31	161	165	15	14	4	3
David Dyke	34	145	140	19	15	4	1
Nick Gray	25	169	167	13	12	3	1
Lynette Hadfield	39	149	147	30	27	5	4
Jane Heywood	33	146	139	13	11	1	1
Teresa Malinowska	27	159	157	20	14	4	3
Liz Parry	29	154	151	22	20	5	3
John Routledge	55	165	163	11	10	2	2
Eileen Ward	27	211	215	40	38	5	4

Victor Burrowes had lost 23 pounds in eleven weeks. He had a sad tale to tell:

> One of the reasons for taking up Fun Runner '82 was excessive weight. Now, 11 weeks into the project my clothes still don't fit me! I shall have to buy a new wardrobe.

What's more, Vic swore that he had not been on a diet. Answering my questionnaire about food, he said that while he was eating less sweets, he was eating more meat, fish, protein, fruit and vegetables. And he continued to enjoy his beer. He also turned out to have a natural talent for running: he entered a three-mile race and came in second in the forty-six-to-fifty age category.

Tim Burton was the 196-pound local government officer who had written to me a few months before. Before starting to exercise he had gone on a semistarvation diet, which he stopped as soon as he started to run. But having dieted, he was weakened, and his fitness level at the start was the lowest of all the men. After eleven weeks he had gained over 4 pounds, but had lost fat.

The most striking example of the way exercise affects body composition rather than weight was Teresa Malinowska, a tall young woman. She had lost a couple of pounds, and was to lose a total of 5 by the end of five months; but in eleven weeks she lost 30 percent of her nonessential body fat. Her body shape changed remarkably. No longer plump, she was lean, and looked radiant.

Jane Heywood started—and ended—the fittest in the group. She was in the habit of cycling to work. Eileen Ward was one of the three very overfat women in the group of sixty-four, none of whom lost weight during the five months of the project, although all lost a small amount of fat. John Routledge showed no change in weight, body fat, or fitness, which was no surprise, because he was not taking any more exercise than he had before. At the beginning of the project his blood pressure, now much lower than the year before, was 144/86. In eleven weeks it came down to 120/80: the blood pressure of a young man.

HOW TO PROLONG YOUR OWN LIFE

While the project was running I heard a doctor say on BBC radio, without a doubt in his voice, that people with high blood pressure usually had to take drugs indefinitely to reduce the pressure. A leaflet put out by the Flora margarine project for heart disease prevention advocates losing weight, eating less salt, and cutting down saturated fats, together with giving up smoking and avoiding tension, as a means to reduce blood pressure. No mention of exercise.

Yet in eleven weeks the blood pressure of the participants fell as follows:

	Before	After
Men	137/93	127/82
Women	127/91	121/82

Dr. Eoin O'Brien and Professor Kevin O'Malley explain the
significance of these figures in their book *High Blood Pressure*. They take the example of a man somewhat older than
most of the men in Fun Runner '82.

> A forty-five-year-old man with a systolic pressure of
> 120 and a diastolic level of 80 may expect to live to
> over 70 years of age. A man of much the same age
> with a systolic pressure of 140 and a diastolic of 95
> may expect to live six years less.

Of the sixty-four who started the five-month project, the
fifteen people with high blood pressure all lowered their
blood pressure by the end, many of them considerably. Here
is the entire list:

		age	Before	After
WOMEN:	age	36	137/95	108/72
		29	134/105	112/80
		29	134/97	113/69
		39	154/111	135/88
		38	132/114	125/81
		29	136/91	117/79
		47	139/98	130/70
		33	138/81	125/75
MEN:	age	46	152/106	130/74
		31	146/91	140/86
		53	158/108	130/90
		25	142/90	135/78
		55	144/86	120/80
		48	140/90	125/66
		26	140/80	122/63

In five months, half a dozen people in their late thirties,
forties or fifties improved their life expectancy by six years.
The man of forty-eight whose blood pressure dropped so
remarkably was Rodney Lewis, a North London taxi driver.
Before the project, he said, he was always pushing his window down and shouting and screaming at silly drivers. His
new blood pressure brought a new personality with it; he lost

his jagged edges and became a calmer man. Vic Burrowes' blood pressure dropped more than 20 points.

Between May and September about ten people dropped out of the project; holidays and other reasons meant that others were not tested three times. Of those who completed the course (and the Fun Run) and were also tested in May, July, and September, the men, on average, lost 9 pounds of body weight and, more significantly, over 20 percent of their nonessential body fat. One man, Tim Burton, gained weight in the five months—all lean tissue. One stayed the same; two kept the same weight but lost fat; the rest lost weight and fat.

The women's results were less striking. On average they lost 4½ pounds of weight and 10 percent of their nonessential fat. The three very overfat women got fitter and completed the two-and-a-half-mile Fun Run to tumultuous cheers; but one did not change her weight or shape much, and the other two actually gained weight, while at the same time losing fat. Paradoxically, they were the two who, at 200 pounds and 211 pounds, would have benefitted most from losing; both were also short in stature. Leaving these three women aside, the rest, half of whom were overweight, half average or slim, lost about 6 pounds in five months.

Losing weight was not, it should be said, a principal reason why people joined the project. In July, halfway through, I asked them all why they had joined, and the most frequently mentioned reasons were "getting fit," "feeling good" and "getting in shape." Defined in this way, the project was a great success for almost everybody who completed it. This table compares the cardiorespiratory fitness of the thirty-four people who completed all the tests, before and after the project.

| | MEN | | WOMEN | |
	Before/after		*Before/after*	
Excellent	1	11	2	6
Good	2	3	4	8
Average	7	0	1	4
Below average	4	0	5	1
Poor	0	0	8	1

EATING WELL—SPONTANEOUSLY

Equally impressive were the comments people made about their eating habits. In July, halfway through, I asked participants how much they were eating, and if they had changed their food habits in any way. Everyone had been strongly advised not to diet in order to keep strength up. Only one person said she was on a diet. If anything, people seemed to be eating more, not less.

I also asked if people were spontaneously eating more or less of different types of food. The only extraneous influence was Audrey Eyton's *F-Plan Diet*, advocating fiber, which became the thing to eat in the summer of 1982. Members of the project were asked to list the types of food they were eating more, or less, of:

Foods	More	Less
Meat and Fish	10	6
Dairy products	9	10
Sugar, sweets, chocolate	7	18
Cereals and pastas	12	7
Fiber	15	1
Alcohol	10	17
Protein	9	3
Fat	0	14
Carbohydrate	9	6
Vitamins	11	2
Fruit	21	2

Replies to questionnaires of this sort must be treated with some caution. Everybody knows that it is a good thing to eat fruit and vegetables, and a bad thing to eat fat, and people no doubt tend to report what they know they ought to do rather than what they actually do. Given this, it was quite striking that ten people said they were drinking more alcohol (usually in the form of beer after runs, judging by the jovial occasions I attended).

The switch away from sugar, sweets and chocolate in favor of cereals and pastas was especially interesting. Sugar and products heavy in sugar are advertised as sources of quick energy, and runners are often (wrongly) told to eat them after a run. By contrast, cereals and pastas have a stodgy image, and people who want to lose weight are often (wrongly) told to avoid them. But the Fun Runners moved away from processed foods—sugars, and also products heavy in sugars and fats—and moved toward whole foods. After eleven weeks of their exercise program, the eating habits of the Fun Runners were approximating the recommendations of the McGovern report, without any prompting from doctors, books or trainers, or from me. Professor Peter Wood of Stanford University tells me he has observed the same spontaneous change in his studies.

HOW TO EAT AS MUCH AS YOU LIKE

The implications of these results are exciting. They suggest that when people become active their bodies tend to prefer foods rich in nourishment that supply energy at a natural rate, and to avoid foods poor in nourishment that supply energy at an unnaturally fast rate. To put it another way, the fit body becomes healthy in part by preferring the foods it needs. For example, one vitamin, thiamine (B_1), is particularly necessary to the active body; and many whole starchy foods are rich in thiamine.

I mentioned these findings to a leading expert on diabetes; for it is now recognized that adult-onset diabetes can be treated by cutting out sugar and by eating whole food rich in starch and fiber. "Ah," he said. "You're one of those people who believes in the wisdom of the body." Yes, I said, I supposed that I was.

On September 26 the members of the project had the time of their lives, running in the *Sunday Times* National Fun Run. A lot of the men had become pretty fast: most of them completed the two-and-a-half-mile course in under eighteen minutes, and Rodney Lewis beat me by a second. The women were less competitive. Debbie Hoyle, a young mother of two children, finished in eighteen minutes and twenty-six seconds; and Cinnia Bermingham, who had written to me five months before saying that she got out of breath running for a bus, finished in nineteen minutes and six seconds. The biggest cheers were for the women in their late thirties and forties, some of whom had developed a fair degree of speed.

The five-month project had accomplished a lot for a good many of the participants. They had lost weight, lost body fat and changed shape. Their blood pressure had come down to the level of young people, and their ability to use oxygen had increased dramatically. They had proved to their own satisfaction that runners are healthy people.

Dr. Barrie Gunter made his own assessment of the project. He said that after twenty-one weeks of exercise the Fun Runners were more self-confident and emotionally stable, more self-assured, more relaxed and composed. He was especially interested in how friendly most people had become. He said:

> My feeling is that this is partly a result of taking part in a group activity with other people all striving towards the same goal; as well as training their bodies, people were also exercising their skills in dealing with other people. The less fit had been helped and encouraged by the more fit.

These benefits are part of what running is all about. Running is, almost uniquely, a social activity, because you can not only run with companions (as opposed to competing against an opponent) but also talk with them while you are running—well, at least until the run becomes a little competitive.

Bill East was fifty-three. At the end of the project his blood pressure had dropped by more than 20 points. He said:

> I have achieved far more than I thought possible. I can run 4½ miles non-stop, my weight, blood pressure and resting heart-rate are all down, and without trying my smoking is down. And I have learned that the body does not deteriorate pro rata with age: I am not that far behind youngsters half my age.

Bill looks ten years younger than he is.

Will Chapman was one of the leaders of the Fun Runner

project. In 1971, weighing 230 pounds, he had a heart attack. Afterward, like John Routledge, he started jogging and became a marathon runner. He said:

> Non-runners ask me what I get out of pounding the streets. My weight is a normal 175 pounds and yet I eat and drink what I want; I'm told I look young for my 45 years and I feel great.

Will was a member of the previous London 1982/50 project, but there is no need to run marathons to benefit from exercise.

Bobbie Randall was forty-seven and the mother of six. "I'm the only fatty left in the family," she explained, writing to join Fun Runner '82. "My job is sedentary, as are my hobbies. I just cannot shift my surplus. Perhaps it's been around too long." In five months she lost 11 pounds, her blood pressure was down from 139/98 to 130/70, her ability to use oxygen had almost doubled, and she ran the Fun Run in twenty-three minutes fifty seconds, coming seventy-first out of 141 in her age category. In January 1983 she won a handicap race of over four miles.

LOSE WEIGHT: EAT MORE

At the time of Fun Runner '82, I was already aware that Professor Peter Wood was mounting similar projects in California with a number of colleagues. Wood, an Englishman who has lived in the United States for twenty years, is deputy director of the Heart Disease Prevention Unit at Stanford, and a veteran of over seventy marathon races. He is also jointly responsible for a nationwide club of veteran joggers and runners, the 50+ Association. Peter Wood's professional specialty is the study of blood lipids, and he is one of the researchers who has found that exercise increases the proportion of beneficial high-density lipoprotein (HDL) in the blood.

In 1976 he mounted a seventeen-week exercise program for twenty-two very overweight women aged between thirty and fifty-two. Most had previously tried and failed to lose weight by dieting. During the program the women also attended classes designed to encourage awareness of their eating habits, but were not told to diet. In practice, most of them made moderate reductions in the amount of food they ate.

At the end of the program, average weight had fallen by 9 pounds. Body fat had decreased by 11 pounds, while lean tissue had increased by 2 pounds. Resting heart rate and heart rate recovery after exercise also decreased, as did blood pressure.

Wood's next projects were more ambitious. He compared the amount of food eaten by sedentary people with that consumed by thirty-four male and twenty-seven female runners aged between thirty-five and fifty-nine, and averaging 35 to 40 miles a week.

As might be expected, the runners were considerably leaner and lighter than the sedentary "control" group. But the runners were eating more—a lot more.

> Male runners consumed 2959 calories a day, vs. 2361 for controls. The corresponding mean values for female runners and controls were 2386 and 1871 calories a day, respectively.

The runners were considerably lighter than the nonrunners, but pound for pound of body weight, they were eating about 50 percent more. Moral: Lose weight, eat more. Gain weight, eat less.

Not everybody wants to run thirty-five to forty miles a week. And sedentary people often assume that the only way to lose weight and fat is to run great distances. However, another study by Peter Wood, of middle-aged women who played ten hours of tennis a week, compared with a control group of sedentary women who on average weighed over 16 pounds more, disproves that. Wood: "We found that the tennis players' food intake was 2417 calories a day, while the overweight women ate only 1490. That's an enormous difference." While not at all huge, the tennis players' energy intake was sufficient to ensure them enough nourishment from vitamins and minerals, given that the food eaten was nutritious. On the other hand, the inactive, overweight women consumed no more energy than many diet books recommend for a semistarvation regime.

The full significance of this pioneering work becomes clear when the energy value of running and playing tennis is measured. Running uses about 9 to 12 calories a minute more than sitting, playing tennis about 5 calories more. Hence the estimate made by Dr. John Garrow that running a marathon consumes about 2500 calories. Hence, also, the notion that you have to walk up and down a mountain to work off the effects of a hearty meal.

The runners studied by Wood were eating 550 calories a day more than the nonrunners. According to the usual calculations, in order to run that extra energy off, at a brisk seven to eight miles an hour, they would have to run for about an hour every day, or fifty to sixty-five miles a week—far more than they were actually running. Even a fast runner would have to do forty-five miles a week to burn off 600 calories a day. Moreover, the runners were lighter than the nonrunners.

The same calculation applied to the tennis players has even more remarkable results. According to the books, you would have to play tennis for 200 minutes a day to burn off 1000 calories, which is twenty-three hours twenty minutes every week. In fact, the tennis players were playing less than half that time. Something is missing from the calculations.

EXERCISE SPEEDS YOU UP

In theory, according to the books, exercise is not a particularly effective way of losing weight and fat. In actual experience, exercise is a most effective way of losing some weight and more fat.

Just as dieting slows you down, exercise of the right type speeds you up. Books recommending exercise usually give charts showing the energy value of different forms of physical activity. But the measurements on which these charts are based, while being accurate as far as they go, do not allow for the fact that certain types of exercise, sustained at a steady intensity for relatively long periods of time, for half an hour or more, speed up the metabolic rate, not only while you are exercising, but also afterward.

As long ago as 1935 it was calculated that vigorous and sustained exercise raises the metabolic rate. This early study estimated that exercise could raise the resting metabolic rate by as much as 25 percent for fifteen hours following the exercise and by perhaps 10 percent for forty-eight hours after that.

The resting metabolic rate of a sedentary woman of average weight has been estimated to account for around 1250 calories a day. In round terms this is one calorie a minute, or 60 calories an hour. Using the figures quoted above, the right kind of exercise, for such a woman, could therefore be worth an extra 15 calories an hour for fifteen hours (equals 225 calories); and an extra 6 calories an hour for forty-eight hours (equals 288 calories). Therefore, in round figures, the true energy value of such exercise could be around 500 calories in addition to the energy used during the exercise.

This, of course, is why the relatively lean women tennis players studied by Professor Wood were eating almost twice as much food as the sedentary—and relatively fat—women.

Any physiologist knows that the metabolic effect of vigorous exercise continues after the exercise has finished. In scientific language, exercise that puts an unusual stress on muscles breaks down muscle fiber (a process termed "catabolism"). The body then rebuilds the muscle fiber ("anabolism") to be stronger and more able to withstand exercise. Repeated exercise, therefore, has a "training effect" and makes one fitter.

Active people know from their own experience that exercise has aftereffects. Stiff muscles, the day after hard exercise, are common and indicate the need for time in which to regenerate. A very common mistake made by people eager to improve their fitness is to exercise daily, on stiff muscles, which then break down further instead of rebuilding. For this reason anyone not an athlete should not, in my view, train hard more than four times a week. The metabolic cycle of catabolism and anabolism (muscle breakdown and buildup) does not of course all happen during the exercise itself.

People who go from a sedentary to an active life enjoy the experience of feeling warmer all the time, because their metabolic rate is higher all the time. Extra body heat is being generated, day and night.

In 1976 the Sports Council of England and Wales commissioned Professor Peter Fentem, a leading British sports physiologist, to prepare a study, "The Case for Exercise." After three years of investigation, one of Dr. Fentem's conclusions was:

> Exercise has a stimulating effect on metabolism which persists throughout the day, raises the metabolic rate and leads to the loss of appreciably more fat than would have been predicted for the exercise undertaken.

In a previous chapter ("Dieting Makes You Fat") it was shown that a lean person may require 300 calories a day more than a fat person of the same weight. Because dieting has the accumulative effect of replacing lean tissue with body fat, the dieter's metabolism slows down. On the other hand, exercise, when vigorous and sustained, has the opposite effect: the more lean tissue people have, the higher their metabolic rate, other things being equal. Exercise has the effect of using body fat as fuel, and at the same time building up lean tissue. The fitter you are, the more you can, and should, eat.

THE RISE OF HOMO SPORTIVUS

The facts that metabolism is dynamic and that exercise using a lot of oxygen speeds up the metabolic rate are so important and basic that people often say to me: "If all this is true, why haven't I heard it before?"

Fit and healthy people tend to be able to do without junk food and drugs; and junk food and drugs are very profitable commodities. That's one, cynical, reason. But there are a number of practical reasons why what is written here is likely to be news to many readers.

The procedure involved in measuring metabolic rate is

complicated and laborious. Far more measurements have been made of changes in metabolic rate as a result of dieting, fasting and overeating than as a result of exercise, simply because it is easier to measure people who are sitting down than to measure them running over a period of months.

Diet books and studies of obesity pay little attention to the role of oxygen because until recently the only people, mountaineers and divers aside, with a direct interest in the relationship of oxygen and energy balance were athletes. Exercise physiology, the science concerned with the effects of oxygen on the human body, was a specialized department, of general interest only to physical education teachers and trainers. Ordinary people take oxygen for granted, just as nutritionists who measure the energy content of food by burning it in a "calorimeter" take it for granted.

The research now being done on exercise and metabolic rate is almost all new, and would have been hard to mount until recently for a very practical reason. Research needs subjects. Until the late 1970s virtually everybody in Western countries remained sedentary throughout life, or else was active only when young. For practical purposes it was unknown for people to get more active as they got older. Professor J. N. Morris, whose studies of London bus conductors and drivers in the 1950s showed that, because they walked up and down the stairs of the double-decker buses, conductors were less likely to suffer heart disease, did his work at a time when doctors commonly believed that exercise was bad for you.

But now the explosion of interest in exercise among ordinary citizens, and in particular the enthusiasm for jogging and running, is turning hundreds of thousands of previously fat people into athletes. Conclusive studies of the effects of exercise on metabolism can be carried out on people who, like the sixty-four Fun Runners, have decided for themselves to progress from being *Homo sedentarius* to *Homo sportivus*.

What is the effect of long-term, regular exercise on metabolic rate, on the quantity and quality of food eaten, on weight, shape, fitness and health? How much exercise is needed to become fit and healthy? Are some forms of exercise better than others? How long should exercise sessions take, and how regular should they be? The Royal College of Physicians' 1983 report on obesity says:

> The physiological effects of short periods of moderately intensive exercise are well defined, and a minimum of 20 minutes of moderate activity three times a week seems sufficient to maintain cardio-vascular responses to physical activity. This degree of activity also seems to play an important role in improving an individual's sense of well-being.

That is to say, a certain type of exercise, carried out with a certain regularity for a certain amount of time, makes you feel good, makes you fit, and makes you healthy. The exercise that produces these effects is now known as "aerobic" exercise.

THE TYPES OF EXERCISE

Dr. Kenneth Cooper is the founding father of the aerobic movement, first in the United States and now throughout the world. In his book *Aerobics* he divides exercise into four types.

Isometrics tense the muscles against themselves or against an immovable object. Isometric exercises strengthen skeletal muscle and are useful for the bedridden and for astronauts. Sometimes they are recommended for executives and office workers who want to do battle with their desks.

Isotonics contract the muscles and also involve movement. As well as strengthening muscle they can make the body either more supple or bulkier. They promote well-being as well as muscular fitness. Examples are the Canadian Air Force exercises, weight training, school physical education and yoga.

Anaerobic exercise divides into two types: either too easy, or too hard, to be aerobic. Literally, "aerobic" means "with oxygen"; and students of exercise have until recently been accustomed to refer to any activity as "aerobic" simply because it uses air. Now, though, the term "aerobic" has come to refer to exercise that makes a sustained demand on the heart and lungs and which uses the big muscles of the body, such as the muscles of the legs.

Anaerobic exercise may be so gentle, or so brief, that it makes no real demands on the heart and the lungs. Alternatively anaerobic exercise may be so intense that after a short while it cannot be sustained; the body cannot supply the volume of oxygen required and goes into "oxygen debt," signaled by severe breathlessness.

Aerobic exercise occupies the middle ground between the two types of anaerobic exercise. It is neither gentle nor intense. It is exercise sustained at a steady, vigorous level for a considerable period of time.

Isometrics and isotonics do not increase the amount of oxygen used by the body, unless they are accompanied by systematic and sustained breathing exercises. Thus, they do not strengthen the heart, lungs and blood vessels.

Any kind of sprinting, whether running, cycling or swimming, is anaerobic, for sprinting cannot be sustained for more than a couple of minutes. What constitutes aerobic activity depends on the state of fitness and health of the individual. A gentle jog may be anaerobic for the fit young person because it is too easy; for the unfit middle-aged person it may be anaerobic because it is too hard.

Dr. Cooper defines aerobic exercise for young people as follows:

> If the exercise is vigorous enough to produce a sustained heart rate of 150 beats a minute or more, the training-effect benefits begin about five minutes after the exercise starts and continue as long as the exercise is performed. If the exercise is not vigorous enough to produce or sustain a heart rate of 150 beats a minute, but is still demanding oxygen, the exercise must be continued considerably longer than five minutes, the total period of time depending on oxygen consumed.

Fitness training may develop physical speed, strength or endurance in different proportions, depending on its purpose. This is true for the Olympic athlete, the patient recovering from a heart attack and for ordinary citizens, whatever their initial level of fitness.

The athlete trains in order to improve performance. A sprinter develops speed rather than endurance; a marathon runner develops endurance rather than strength. Exercise that develops strength or speed but not endurance is anaerobic. Exercise that develops endurance is aerobic, because endurance is achieved by training the body's capacity to use oxygen. Aerobic exercise promotes health through fitness because, by its sustained use of oxygen, it strengthens the heart, lungs, blood vessels and other vital organs, as well as the muscles.

This is why, as Dr. Cooper states, in order to be aerobic, exercise must elevate the heart rate past a certain point for a certain period of time. The reason sprinting is anaerobic is that it uses oxygen stored within the muscle itself, which is soon exhausted. On the other hand, jogging (at a speed appropriate to the physical condition of the individual) is aerobic, because it uses oxygen breathed in from the air.

WHAT IS "AEROBIC" EXERCISE?

Doctors and scientists specializing in the heart and in exercise physiology have determined that to be aerobic, exercise must be sustained for at least five minutes, preferably for ten; and that during this time the heart rate should rise to 60 to 80 percent of its maximum capacity. Below the 60 percent level, exercise will not strengthen the cardiovascular system. And only exceptionally fit people can gain aerobic benefit from exercise above the 80 percent level.

Some men (it's almost always men) push themselves too hard on exercise programs, and there is even a condition known as "positive addiction": the jogger who cannot do without the daily session. I see nothing but good in running a lot if you enjoy it; but as I have previously said, I always advise people, including runners training for marathons, to run no more than four times a week.

Progress in running and other aerobic activities is much like progress in any other area of life: it goes by fits and starts. You reach a certain level, then stick on this "plateau" for a while, sometimes quite a long time; then there is a "breakthrough" to a higher level. It's important not to expect progress to be steady. Many training programs make that mistake.

Here are the most common questions people ask me about aerobic exercise. First: "Which sports and activities are aerobic and which are anaerobic?" Second: "How can I discover when my heart rate is elevated to 60 to 80 percent of maximum?" Third: "How long should I exercise each day and each week?" Fourth: "How long will it take for the exercise to have a good effect on my health?"

AN EXERCISE PROGRAM TO FOLLOW

The "Health Through Fitness" schedule on pages 189–91 is a guide to an aerobic exercise program that any able-bodied person can follow and is designed to take the mystery out of aerobic exercise.

If you can, join your local jogging club or aerobics class. If you have any doubts about your health, see your physician and explain that you are about to take regular exercise. If your physician thinks that exercise is unhealthy, insist on seeing a doctor who agrees with exercise. The modern view is that you do not need medical "clearance" to exercise if you are able-bodied and under sixty years old. A sedentary life is much more dangerous. The advantage of joining a jogging club or aerobics class is that you should then have access not only to experienced people who can guide you but also to doctors expert in the treatment of fit and healthy people as opposed to ill people. Motivation is the special advantage of a club or group: everybody in the Fun Runner '82 project agreed that the spirit of the teams furnished added incentive to keep going.

In answer to the first question, there is almost no such thing as an intrinsically aerobic or anaerobic sport or activity. It all depends on how the game is played and on the condition of the player. Because it is too leisurely, baseball is an out-door sport involving activity that is bound to be anaerobic. Other sports, such as football, hockey, basketball and squash, are aerobic only if played rather eccentrically, in continuous movement. Men who bring their competitive urges to the squash court and flail around, imagining that sweat and exhaustion are proof against the excesses of their everyday lives, are making a mistake. Squash played that way is anaerobic and will develop speed and strength but not endurance. Played fast, it is safe only for the highly fit person; played sporadically by someone with a sedentary job, it is fairly dangerous. Tennis and badminton, if played with some skill, are more likely to be aerobic.

By their nature, judo, boxing, karate and yoga are unlikely to be aerobic. Working out in a gymnasium and downhill skiing can only be aerobic for the exceptionally fit person who can keep going without stopping for ten minutes. If you are a recreational skier you may imagine that you can regularly ski for ten minutes or more without a break. Next time you are on the slopes, time yourself. Weight training can be aerobic only if carried out on special equipment such as Nautilus machines.

The recreations most likely to be aerobic are brisk walking, preferably in hilly country, and dancing. "Aerobics," sometimes called "aerobic dancing," is a form of vigorous dancing specifically planned for continuous ten-minute sessions. Golf can be an aerobic exercise for older people, because of the distances walked between shots. If a golf cart is used the sport cannot be aerobic.

The best aerobic exercise is any exercise that can be sustained for ten minutes or more at a time. Jogging may be the "best" aerobic exercise simply because it is cheap, convenient and possible virtually any day of the year. (For the beginner, a combination of walking and jogging will be aerobic; for a more experienced person, running.) Bicycling is aerobic only if you are able to keep going without stops. Traffic lights defeat the purpose, whereas a long ride in the countryside can be good aerobic exercise. Swimming is better all-around exercise, because it uses the whole body. The disadvantages of swimming are practical: access to pools, crowds, chlorine, the difficulty of swimming for ten minutes or more without a break. Cross-country skiing is the best aerobic exercise of all, and champion cross-country skiers have the highest aerobic capacity of all sportsmen and women.

A sedentary person who is out of condition, perhaps overweight, and middle-aged, with a history of breathlessness may at first find any sport or formal exercise too hard; even brisk walking may be quite taxing. Someone in this condition would certainly be out of breath walking up flights of stairs. If this describes you, be patient! Go for walks of ten minutes and more at your own pace, and don't think of taking vigorous exercise until you feel ready. As the members of Fun Runner '82 discovered, the body is remarkably resilient and develops quite quickly in response to exercise.

MEASURING HEART RATE

The second question I am most often asked is "How can I discover when my heart rate is elevated to 60 to 80 percent of maximum?" Dr. Cooper's estimate of 150 beats a minute applies to younger people, because maximum heart rate is a function of age. Roughly speaking, maximum rate is 220 beats a minute minus your age. For example, at the time of writing I am forty-four years old, so my maximum rate is 176 beats a minute: that is about as fast as my heart will go. Thus younger people have faster maximum rates than older people.

The way to find out whether you are exercising aerobically is to take your pulse, immediately after exercise, at the wrist or if you prefer at the neck, using a watch with a second hand.

This drill is a feature of every well-organized aerobics class. Remember that the exercise should take five minutes at the very minimum: increase it to ten minutes or more as soon as you can. It is best to take your pulse for ten seconds the moment you stop exercising and then multiply by six. Heart rates for people of different ages are as follows:

Age	Maximum rate (minute)	60 to 80% rate (minute)	60 to 80% rate (10 seconds)
under 25	200	120–160	20–27
25–29	195	117–156	20–26
30–34	190	114–152	19–25

Age	Maximum rate (minute)	60 to 80% rate (minute)	60 to 80% rate (10 seconds)
35–39	185	111–148	19–25
40–44	180	108–144	18–24
45–49	175	105–140	18–23
50–54	170	102–136	17–23
55–59	165	99–132	17–22
60–64	160	96–128	16–21
65 and over	155	93–124	16–21

There are two other ways of determining whether the exercise you're doing is aerobic. However, since neither involves a watch or taking the pulse, they are less precise. The "perceived effort" test (also called the "Borg scale" because it was developed by Gunnar Borg at the University of Stockholm) requires practice and some self-knowledge, to rate the exercise you do on a scale of 6 to 20:

6		14	
7	very, very light	15	hard
8		16	
9	very light	17	very hard
10		18	
11	fairly light	19	very, very hard
12		20	
13	somewhat hard		

Aerobic exercise should feel "somewhat hard" or "hard," corresponding to 12 to 16 on the scale. You can verify your judgment by checking to see if it relates to a heart rate of roughly 120 to 160 beats a minute. With practice, it is easy to judge without a watch that light or very hard exercise is not aerobic.

The third way of checking whether exercise is aerobic is the "talk test," which is most useful during a jog. During aerobic exercise you should be able to carry on a conversation, even if in somewhat staccato fashion. If you cannot talk during exercise then it cannot be aerobic and will be ineffective; it means your heart rate is likely to have soared well above 150 beats a minute and you will be in "oxygen debt," with the result that you will have to slow down to an aerobic level of exercise, or stop.

Unfit people often worry unnecessarily about the possible dangers of exercise. The body has ways of foiling people who try too hard. Exhaustion is its first defense. Anybody who persists in exercising too hard is likely to get injured or depressed. "Jogger's blues" is a well-known condition that results from following a training program designed for an athlete, not an ordinary citizen. Injuries should always be seen as a helpful warning sign. Do not continue to exercise if the pain of an injury gets worse or if the pain is sharp. In such cases see a sympathetic doctor.

To some extent aerobic exercise can be built into your life. Walk to work or to the station; walk up stairs; cycle to work. Some of the women who graduated from the London 1982/50 and later projects now run to work and have insisted on the installation of showers.

HOW MUCH EXERCISE?

The third and fourth questions I am most often asked are "How long should I exercise, each day and each week?" and "How long will it take for the exercise to improve my health?"

Strictly speaking, the answer to the fourth question is "It depends." The exercise programs for which I have been responsible—London 1982/50, Fun Runner '82 and, later, the *Sunday Times* Getting in Shape and the Sisters projects—have lasted between five months and a year. The most remarkable changes in all these projects happened about three months after the training began. Men and women of different ages found that their shapes changed (as measured by estimates of body fat, a better gauge than body weight); that they slept better and often needed less sleep; that they enjoyed eating and drinking what they liked; that they gained a natural sense of well-being (and were less inclined to continue with a course of drugs or psychoanalysis); and that they were recovering an enjoyment of their bodies and of playing and striving with other people that they assumed they had lost at the end of childhood.

I asked some participants to tell me what had happened. Michael Innes, a relatively fit twenty-eight-year-old, reported:

> Running represents a personal challenge. Eight weeks on from the first tentative steps there has been no great metamorphosis; just a feeling of well-being and a remedy, perhaps, for mental fatigue after a day's work.

Terry Bennett, a forty-one-year-old solicitor who lost nearly 30 pounds, observed:

> I love those magic mornings when a mile into the run you feel good, and you know this is a day when you can push yourself almost to your limit for mile after mile, and you finish physically tired but mentally exhilarated.

He was writing about runs in winter, before breakfast and a day's work. Peter Bird, a fifty-seven-year-old insurance underwriter and a veteran of several marathons, had been a diabetic who some years before had decided to save his own life by running. He wrote, of a time when he was 55 pounds heavier:

> I used to roll off the train at Charing Cross in the morning feeling dizzy with the high blood pressure. I honestly believe that if I hadn't been encouraged to run, seven years ago, I would be dead by now.

Liz Parry, a twenty-nine-year-old teacher training, not for a marathon, but for the Fun Run, wrote:

> I am frankly amazed that I am improving in ways that I thought were personally impossible.

Vivienne Coady, married to a club athlete, enjoyed winning at her own level:

> Once we have put in a couple of miles, I feel really great. I never feel tired; rather, a feeling of being refreshed. When I have felt tired before the run, I no longer feel so, afterwards.

She became a trainer for the *Sunday Times* Getting in Shape project as a way of giving to others what she had got herself. Don Clark, a forty-one-year-old probation officer, ran for another reason, to raise £10,000 for another machine like the one that had saved his life: a long operation had disentangled a cyst from his spinal column. He ran not to save his own life, but those of others. He found:

> Running is peaceful, and it represents a kind of freedom. It establishes warm bonds between people. Part of me fell in love with the hippy ideal in the 1960s. The best parts of running allow me to relive the best parts of that.

The reply I enjoyed most came from James Kelly, a forty-nine-year-old local government officer from Swansea:

> I felt lethargic and content to let life pass me by. Then in 1978 I joined in the first *Sunday Times* National Fun Run. Suddenly I was no longer one of life's spectators. Even the youngest typist was no longer looking at me as if I were her father. Success at last!

People who diet want to stop. People who persevere with an exercise program do not want to stop.

HOW LONG SHOULD YOU EXERCISE?

Experts broadly agree. Dr. Cooper and Professor Wood have found that lasting health benefits occur at 80 to 120 minutes of exercise a week, preferably in four sessions. For a jogger this is the equivalent of a total of a gentle eight to twelve miles a week, covered perhaps on two days during the week and the two weekend days, the sessions being as evenly spaced as possible. At this level profound changes in the cardiorespiratory system start and continue.

The U.S. Health and Social Services Secretary Richard Schweiker, who had served as a member of the McGovern committee in 1977, said in 1981:

> By taking five simple steps, by not smoking, by using alcohol in moderation, by eating a proper diet and getting the proper amount of exercise and sleep, a forty-five-year-old man can expect to live ten or eleven years longer than a person who does not make these choices.

The hundreds of people of all ages I have run with, talked to and corresponded with in the last five years have taught me that exercise should be the first one of these five steps. The others follow as a result of the exercise. And "proper diet" turns out to have nothing whatever to do with dieting: for most people who exercise regularly, a proper diet is eating as much good food as they want to eat.

MORE OXYGEN; MORE FOOD

Why is aerobic exercise so special? First of all, because it speeds up the body and increases our metabolic rate. Doctors and scientists who have not found that exercise produces this effect have not studied aerobic exercise.

We need oxygen for our internal fire that burns food. The more oxygen that is supplied to a flame, the brighter and faster the flame burns; this is as true within the human body as it is within a grate. The action of a bellows fans a fire; the action of the lungs, themselves a form of bellows, sends oxygen into the bloodstream for use in the conversion of food into energy.

The analogy with a fire in a grate is fair. Suitably ventilated, a small amount of coal burns bright and low; a large amount of coal burns bright and high. If a bellows is applied to a small amount of coal, more will soon be needed. If, on the other hand, little air can get to either a small or a large amount of coal, it will burn low, or not be burned at all.

The greater a person's capacity for oxygen, the higher the metabolic rate of that person will be. The more oxygen that is supplied, the more food the body can burn. To be more precise, there is a relationship between the oxygen intake of a person and the volume of food he or she requires, in order to be in energy balance. The more fuel, the bigger the fire.

The reason that the metabolic rate of the person on a diet or a fast goes down is not a mystery. The body balances a reduced food intake by reducing oxygen intake, and reduces oxygen intake still more when energy has to be taken not from food but from the body itself. Dieters train their bodies to require less oxygen. The main effect of diet regimes is to condition the body to tolerate diets, which it does by lowering its metabolic rate, which is to say its use of oxygen. The more frequent and the more stringent the diet regimes, the more dramatic and less reversible these effects will be.

It also follows that the body will balance a greater intake of food by taking in more oxygen, up to the point at which it has no more capacity. A very big man who is also phenomenally physically active will therefore have a gigantic appetite, but when as a result of change of habits or age or infirmity he ceases to exercise, much of the food he eats will turn to fat. Hence the dramatic fattening of Henry VIII and Edward VII when they stopped hunting.

In addition to the food it takes in, the body contains another fuel: fat. Just as food is burned with oxygen, fat is burned with oxygen. Because dieting lowers the body's capacity for oxygen, it also lowers the body's capacity to burn its own fat, which is stored, instead.

To sum up: when energy from food outbalances energy from oxygen, fat is stored, and obesity is the result. Because dieting reduces energy from oxygen, it is self-defeating. Overeating increases the use of oxygen, but is outbalanced by the extra energy taken in from food. The way out of this vicious circle is to use more fuel: to apply the bellows of the lungs to the body's fire.

THE MUSCLE THAT USES FAT AS FUEL

Sustained aerobic exercise results in loss of fat and gain of lean tissue. In time its "training effect" increases the metabolic activity of the muscles at all times. Another reason why aerobic rather than anaerobic exercise has this effect is that the two types of exercise use different types of muscle. There are two kinds of muscle fiber: red muscle fiber (also known as "slow-twitch" muscle), used for work requiring endurance; and white muscle fiber (also known as "fast-twitch" muscle), used for work requiring immediate reaction. Aerobic exercise uses red muscle, anaerobic exercise white muscle.

It is not known to what extent, if at all, exercise can alter the proportions of red and white muscle. It is known that some people are "red muscle types," meaning that their muscles contain a relatively high proportion of red fibers; and other people are "white muscle types," their muscles containing a relatively high proportion of white fibers. Take runners as an example: sprinters are white muscle types, constantly using fast-twitch fiber for explosive action; marathoners are red muscle types, constantly using slow-twitch fiber for their methodical long-distance running.

The fuel used by white muscle fiber is glycogen—naturally enough, because glycogen is the body's immediately available source of energy, and can be instantly mobilized. The glycogen store is essential, and together with the water bound up with it, must be replaced after the white muscle fibers have done their anaerobic work. Anaerobic activity does not burn fat. This is why it is physically impossible to lose fat, or indeed to lose weight, except temporarily, if your style of playing squash is to thrash around the court anaerobically.

Red muscle fiber also uses glycogen as fuel. But, to take the analogy of a domestic fire, it does so not as its main fuel, but as kindling. The main fuel for red muscle is body fat, which, like coal, is slow-burning and releases great energy. To be more precise, red muscle fiber uses fat released from the body's stores into the bloodstream, in the form of a liquid, free fatty acid. The fat store of the body is, of course, there to be used as fuel, and unlike glycogen does not need to be replaced.

It is aerobic exercise—endurance work—that uses red muscle, and hence fat, as fuel. This is common sense. Aerobic exercise corresponds to the work done by people who do not live in industrialized societies, such as Eskimos and Bushmen; or remote people such as Lapps; or peasants in the West, such as the country people of the Swiss Alps. These people work aerobically and eat well and generally go through life without getting fat. It is constant walking that keeps them lean.

Just like any machine that is neglected and rusted, the function of the human body degenerates with disuse. Sedentary adults who fondly imagine that it is only dignity that prevents them gamboling about as they did when children should have a try when no one is looking: they will have an unpleasant surprise.

A machine that is carefully tended and oiled will preserve its usefulness. Here, though, the human body is unlike a machine: for the body actually improves with use. This is conspicuously the case with muscle.

Muscles need oxygen. Aerobic training develops the flow of oxygen within muscle, and this in turn develops the functioning of the muscle. In particular, the "training effect" created by three to six months' aerobic exercise (for most able-bodied people) develops the ability of muscle to use fat as fuel. The human body is marvelously responsive to the positively beneficial stress put upon it by regular, vigorous exercise.

Conversely, it is idle to suppose that muscle will remain in good shape if, after childhood, the body becomes inactive. Our bodies are in a state of constant modification, throughout life. The muscle fiber of sedentary people becomes increasingly shot through with fat, just like the marbled steak from a steer kept artificially penned up, so as to provide juicy, fatty meat.

IS THERE HOPE FOR VERY FAT PEOPLE?

The muscle fiber of sedentary people, who use less and less oxygen, adjusts so as to use less and less oxygen. Thus, sedentary people gradually lose the wherewithal for burning fat. Some new evidence suggests that, with long disuse, red muscle degenerates into white-type muscle, compounding the problem. If this is so, it explains why doctors who work with very obese patients state that exercise is ineffective as a means of weight control. It also explains why the three very overweight women who completed the Fun Runner '82 project got fitter but, paradoxically, did not lose weight and lost little fat.

Experienced and conscientious doctors who work with grossly obese patients more often than not form the view—privately, if not publicly—that obesity is intractable. Jaw-wiring, or semistarvation regimes in hospital conditions, over a period of perhaps a year achieve massive weight loss. But, as with "Weight Watcher of the Year" or "Slimmer of the Year" contests, most very obese people who lose remarkable amounts of weight regain it, and more, in time.

It is possible that some very obese people have indeed irreversibly lost the ability to use fat as fuel. There comes a point with various diseases and disorders when damage cannot be reversed. Faced with the choice of surgery or philosophy, the wise choice is, like Falstaff, to make the best of a big and burgeoning body.

But it is probable that the majority of people who are overfat, even very overfat, can reverse their state by means of exercise. First, one must understand that the process by which the naturally active body of childhood turns to fat when adult and sedentary is a slow, long process, not reversible in a week or a month. Moreover, replacing relatively inactive fat with active lean tissue will discourage those who rely on their bathroom scales, because muscle is heavier than fat. As you start to exercise and so regenerate your body, the measurement to take is of your waist, not your weight. And be patient!

If your purpose in exercising is not only to become fit, but also to lose fat, there is increasing evidence that the secret is not intensity, but duration, of exercise. Dr. Eric Newsholme of Oxford University, a biochemist who is currently working on new research on this subject, is inclined to believe that the body contains what might be termed a "fat-burning mechanism" which is switched on only after maybe half an hour of exercise.

If Dr. Newsholme is right, and my own experience and that of the people I have worked with suggests that he is, then the motto for people who want to lose fat is: keep going. My recommendation for sedentary, out-of-shape adults, especially if over thirty-five, is long walks, first of all. If they are vigorous enough to work up a sweat, these walks will be aerobic; and if they last half an hour or more, with no stops, in three months or so—sometimes sooner—they will be good for the waistline.

THE VALUE OF WALKING

The new enthusiasm for jogging and running, which I share, may have the unfortunate effect, for some people, of discouraging them from taking less vigorous—and less conspicuous—forms of exercise. Citizens do not get medals for walking—even for the marathon distance of twenty-six and more miles—but if your purpose, in taking exercise, is to lose fat, it may very well be that the most effective method is to walk long distances rather than to run for a couple of miles. And walking, especially in the countryside on weekends, can be a way to enjoy fresh air and the company of your family, or at least your dog.

I foresee a time when health centers are established throughout Western countries, with the purpose of encouraging citizens to realize their full potential, by means of health tests followed by individual advice on food and exercise. Meanwhile, long vigorous walks will not only trim your waistline, but also enliven the functions of your gut and encourage a sense of natural well-being.

What about hunger? Many people are put off by exercise

because they find that afterward they feel ravenously hungry. Writers who favor exercise tend to claim that, for reasons which are unclear to them, exercise does not make you hungry. My experience is that most people who take exercise scoff at such claims; most exercise makes you hungry, all right. So how can exercise lead to weight loss?

Remember that aerobic exercise speeds up your metabolic rate throughout the day. After a while you will notice that difference: you will wear fewer clothes, take blankets off the bed and sleep with a window open, stop suffering from cold hands and feet, and generally feel warmer all the time. That's what having a higher metabolic rate means, in terms of everyday experience. So don't worry about feeling hungry. Eat! The secret, though, is to eat whole, bulky foods, full of nourishment, and to lay off foods saturated with processed sugars and fats. There are few meals more satisfying than a steaming hot vegetable stew, with meat too if you like, on the day of a long walk or run. My own favorite is ratatouille. Oxtail also makes a delicious stew.

Remember, too, that aerobic exercise loses fat and gains lean tissue. You may, or may not, lose weight, but don't worry about it. Instead, measure your waistline (and other parts of your body, as shown on page 193). Enjoy a little ceremony: burn all the calorie charts you have in the house, and then put your bathroom scales in the trash.

HOW TO BURN YOUR OWN FAT

Dr. Newsholme's investigations may, however, explain why some physiologists have found that exercise may not make you hungry. The fitter you are, and the more exercise you take, the more your body is trained, during aerobic exercise, to burn its own fat. But exercise taking less than half an hour, whether or not it is aerobic, will mostly use glycogen as fuel. And since hunger is signaled when glycogen stores are low, it follows that an exercise of any type lasting under half an hour will have the effect of making you hungry; whereas relatively gentle exercise, if longer-lasting, will use body fat and will not make you hungry.

This hypothesis certainly corresponds with my own experience. For me, a short run of four miles makes me hungry; whereas after a long weekend run of maybe fifteen miles, lasting two hours or more, I do not feel like a meal. Moreover, I have often noticed a "third wind" after thirty to forty minutes into a run, which might be the fat-burning mechanism "switching on." Dr. Newsholme's proposals are backed by his own experience of progressing from a sedentary 230-pounder to a 175-pound marathon runner. It will take a number of years before some of the most exciting scientific work being done in the fields of food and exercise can be validated. Meanwhile, good advice to anyone who has decided to become fit and healthy is to trust your own experience.

Aerobic exercise is the most effective treatment for the most common disorders of the gut. I have never come across a constipated jogger. It's my opinion, too, that aerobic exercise is the most effective first step to positive health, because, as with the Fun Runner '82 members, regular exercise brings with it an appetite for good whole food. I have lost count of the number of people, who now take regular exercise, who have said to me: "I really used to look forward to cream buns and doughnuts and chocolate eclairs—but now, I may think I fancy them, but I don't." My own version of this experience was the first time I ran eighteen miles: four circuits of Hyde Park and Kensington Gardens in London. The last lap was very painful, and I only kept going by thinking of the fudge ice cream and coffee eclairs I'd soon devour as my reward. As it turned out, I threw these treats away; I couldn't stomach them. They were too sweet, too "rich."

If aerobic exercise indeed damps down the desire for processed sugar, then it must be vital in preventing and treating diabetes. That is the view of Professor Michael Berger, a leading specialist in diabetes. Any diabetic whose pancreas is destroyed will of course have to go on injecting insulin. But almost all diabetics, including children, have a pancreas which is damaged but not destroyed; and Dr. Berger has found that his patients respond to regular exercise. Indeed, he has found that diabetic children, who are often told that exercise is dangerous, are at risk not from the exercise, but from the amount of insulin they inject, which becomes an overdose when combined with exercise. The solution is to exercise and lower the dose of insulin.

The way, therefore, to prevent or alleviate adult-onset diabetes is to exercise and eat good food. There comes a point in any severe disease when it is irreversible; before that, however, it can be reversed, or at least allayed, simply by using the body well. In the case of diabetes, the best means to mend and nourish the pancreas is to allow it to restore its natural function, by eating whole food rich in protein, essential fats, fiber, vitamins and minerals, and no processed sugars.

Many modern doctors, scientists and therapists have come to realize that in the long view, the prescription for the prevention and treatment of Western diseases is exactly the same as the Rx for positive health: plenty of fresh air and plenty of good food. It is only our fascination with technology that prevents us from practicing what doctors down the ages always knew.

A STRONG HEART, A LIVELY BODY

The effects of aerobic exercise on the function of the heart, lungs and blood vessels are well known. With sustained aerobic exercise, say for sessions totaling 80 to 120 minutes a week, the blood vessels enlarge and become more elastic. The heart, itself a muscle, becomes stronger and larger. Blood pressure drops. A further consequence is that resting heart rate drops, from, say, the "average" 72 beats a minute or more, to 60 and then down even further, to maybe 50.

Trained athletes often have a heart rate in the 40s. The average heart rate of the London 1982/50 participants dropped to the 50s after marathon training. The simplest test for a healthy heart is resting heart rate; and it is very satisfying, knowing this, to find that heart rate drops, steadily, during a course of aerobic training.

At the same time, the heart also pumps more blood. Dr. Kenneth Cooper estimates that aerobically trained people will have up to two extra pints of blood in their bodies. This is because of a process of "vascularization" whereby blood vessels not only enlarge but also grow in number. The blood vessels on the surface of the heart itself become larger and more elastic, and are therefore far less likely to be the site of a heart attack. Thomas Bassler, an American doctor, has claimed that running marathons gives anyone without a pre-existing heart condition 100 percent protection against a fatal heart attack caused by irreversible blockage within a blood vessel. This claim is disputed, but there is no doubt that a runner's cardiovascular system is stronger than that of a nonrunner.

It is healthier as well as stronger. Professor Wood, supported by other studies, has shown that high proportions of the abrasive, useful HDL lipoprotein are associated with aerobic exercise, equivalent to jogging eight to twelve miles a week. Below that level, exercise does not have a great effect on lipid levels. In California, where anyone can buy a customized car registration number, Professor Wood's is HIGH HDL, to remind people in the car behind of the good effects of running.

Aerobic exercise also promotes the growth of blood vessels close to the surface of the skin. This accounts for the healthy glow of runners and encourages rejuvenation of the skin. There is also evidence that aerobic exercise slows down or even reverses the tendency of bone to decalcify and grow brittle with age. Old people who break their bones as a result of a fall are usually sedentary people. According to the Royal College of Physicians, echoing experts in the United States:

> The need for middle-aged and elderly people to continue to engage in regular and substantial periods of moderate activity each week runs counter to current practice. . . . There seems little doubt that the majority of adults in sedentary occupations are physiologically "unfit" with poor cardiovascular responses to exercises.

REASONS FOR THE EXERCISE "HIGH"

New research is being done on the relationship of aerobic exercise to endorphin levels. Only recently identified, endorphins are chemical substances whose structure is similar to morphine. Consequently they are sometimes known as "the body's natural opiates." There is some evidence that endorphin pathways are the pathways traced by acupuncturists, and so account for the otherwise mysterious anesthetic effect of acupuncture.

Endorphins are released by the body under induced stress, like exercise, and may postpone the sensation of pain in physical crisis until the need for action has passed. They may be what enables a footballer with a broken collarbone to score a goal, or a runner with blisters to complete a race.

There is evidence that smoking inhibits the flow of endorphins, replacing this natural process with the artificial comfort of nicotine; hence smoking's addictive qualities. There is also evidence that aerobic exercise "jogs" the endorphins into action. So the way to stop smoking may be not to try to give it up, but to start aerobic exercise, and see what happens. Half the London 1982/50 and Fun Runner '82 participants who started as smokers found that they stopped more or less spontaneously during the projects, as they found themselves enjoying the "jogger's high," the natural and intense sense of well-being of which endorphins are the source. Hence Terry Bennett's "magic mornings."

For people who are out of shape, aerobic exercise is the way forward. We need more air. Aerobic exercise allows us to eat more while losing fat, whereas dieting will only depress an overweight person. Aerobics puts the body in energy balance at a natural level so that good food can provide enough nourishment. Aerobic exercise enlivens the alimentary tract and strengthens the cardiovascular system. It is the means to health through fitness.

HEALTH THROUGH FITNESS

The following aerobic training schedule is based on ten rules, seven stages, and forty-nine steps to be taken at your own pace. It will work for all able-bodied people whatever their initial state of fitness. Remember that it takes a long time for the body to get out of shape; so it will take some months to regain what you have lost.

THE TEN RULES

1. *Start at the beginning.* Whatever your initial state of fitness, start at stage 1. Do not move up a stage until you can comfortably complete every session in a week.
2. *Variety is the spice.* Some sessions are longer, others are shorter; the longer sessions last ten minutes in stage 1 and increase to forty minutes in stage 7. The short sessions build from five to ten minutes to twenty to thirty minutes.
3. *Rest as well as exercise.* Start with three and then four sessions a week, as shown, with rest days in between. (The chart assumes that weekend days are convenient; if not, of course, other days will do as well.)
4. *One step and stage at a time.* Progress at your own pace. Don't force yourself to move from one stage to the next. The best test of your progress is a sense of well-being and energy after you exercise.
5. *Backsliding is OK.* If you find a stage too hard, move back. If you get fed up or ill for a while, don't worry. Start a stage below where you left off. You will enjoy holidays more if you keep exercising.
6. *Train aerobically.* Walk-jogging, then jogging, is the most reliable aerobic exercise: it is simple, available, easy to measure. The two longer sessions should be jogging. For the other sessions, please yourself with any aerobic exercise.
7. *Measure your own fitness.* At the very beginning, and every time you move up a stage, measure your fitness (by means of the system on page 192).
8. *First target is 80 to 120 minutes a week.* Stages 5–7 are where the cardiovascular benefits will take place, provided that your exercise is aerobic.
9. *Second target is eight to twelve miles a week.* As soon as you reach stage 5, you are ready for the "two-mile" test on page 192. Use this to check that you are, when you jog, covering eight to twelve miles a week or the equivalent in other aerobic exercise.
10. *Warm up and warm down.* Before and after every session,

stretch and bend your body, and jog on the spot or walk for a few minutes.

There is no rule about how long it will take to reach stage 5; it all depends on you. If you treat the schedule as a competition and push yourself through the stages, you are fairly likely to injure yourself. As a rough guide, the majority of people I have worked with have taken ten to twenty weeks to reach stage 5.

THE SEVEN STAGES AND THE 49 STEPS

	Sat.	Sun.	Mon.	Tues.	Wed.	Thurs.	Fri.	Total
Stage 1	*10*	—	—	*5*	—	5	—	20
Stage 2	*15*	—	—	*5*	—	10	—	30
Stage 3	*20*	—	—	*10*	—	10	—	40
Stage 4	*25*	10	—	*10*	—	15	—	60
Stage 5	*30*	15	—	*15*	—	20	—	80
Stage 6	*35*	15	—	*25*	—	25	—	100
Stage 7	*40*	20	—	*30*	—	30	—	120

Days printed in bold are the days for jogging. If you prefer to jog on all three or four days a week, that's fine. If not, check that the exercise on the other one or two days really is aerobic. All days left blank are rest days. The rest days are a vital part of the forty-nine steps. The numbers refer to minutes. As long as the total for the week is right, you can vary the length of any session, but do not shorten the long run and do not cut out sessions.

This schedule is designed to give you a framework, but you can design a schedule to suit yourself. Just make sure that your own schedule follows the ten rules above.

You may well want to base your own schedule on aerobics classes. If these classes are really and truly aerobic, then include them as part of your schedule. But often "aerobics" classes are not really aerobic: test them. In any case, don't rely completely on classes. In the long term the most effective aerobic exercise is vigorous walking, graduating to jogging and running, simply because this exercise is readily sustained at a steady 60–80 percent of maximum heart rate.

MEASURING YOUR OWN FITNESS

The sense of physical and mental well-being that grows with aerobic exercise is as good an indication of the development of health through fitness as any test a physician can perform.

You will find it valuable and fascinating to measure the development of your health through fitness. Use the tests on page 193 every time you reach a new stage in the seven-stage plan.

The "self-measurement" tests on the chart you can carry out yourself. The way to measure your heart rate at rest and after exercise is explained on page 174. The "fitness tests" are offered at some health clubs and doctors' clinics. Search them out.

When you reach stage 5, find out how long it takes you to run two miles. Eight laps of an athletic track is near enough two miles; otherwise prepare a route on a large-scale map. Do the two-mile test every month once you reach stage 5.

Gear. You will need shoes especially made for jogging. These have built-up heels and look a bit like landing craft. They are expensive. Do not skimp on them; they prevent injuries to the lower legs and knees. You will also need a track suit for cold days, and of course shorts and T-shirts.

Diary. You will find it very helpful to keep a diary in which you enter every exercise session, together with notes on the weather, your state of health at the time, how you felt, length of exercise session, and so on. As time goes on and you get fitter, a diary is great for motivation, and as a means to pay attention to your body. You might like to make copies of the self-measurement tests and insert them in your diary.

Clubs and classes. Jogging clubs that welcome beginners have sprung up everywhere. Aerobics classes are also growing at a great rate. Clubs or classes are great for motivation, and can be good fun too. Find one in your locality by consulting the local Y, or even, in some enlightened cities, city hall.

Magazines. The specialist magazines, most of which are new, regularly carry details of clubs, classes, new ideas, fitness testing centers, and so forth. For the jogger and runner the magazines are *The Runner* and *Runner's World*. For everybody with an interest in fitness, health and good food, the magazine is *American Health*.

SELF-MEASUREMENT

Start Stages:

	1	2	3	4	5	6	7
Body (inches)							
Chest/Bust	__	__	__	__	__	__	__
Waist	__	__	__	__	__	__	__
Hips	__	__	__	__	__	__	__
Thighs	__	__	__	__	__	__	__
Weight (pounds)	__	__	__	__	__	__	__
Heart rate (per minute)							
At rest	__	__	__	__	__	__	__
After exercise[1]	__	__	__	__	__	__	__
3 minutes after	__	__	__	__	__	__	__
10 minutes after	__	__	__	__	__	__	__
Two-mile test							
Minutes/seconds taken					__	__	__
Fitness tests (to be professionally administered)							
Blood pressure	__	__	__	__	__	__	__
Body fat percentage	__	__	__	__	__	__	__
Oxygen capacity[2]	__	__	__	__	__	__	__
Fitness rating[3]	__	__	__	__	__	__	__

1. Immediately afterwards.
2. Vo$_2$ Max (ml O$_2$ min kg).
3. Cooper scales.

The charts and schedule on these pages were designed in consultation with Will Chapman, Dr. Kenneth Cooper, Malcolm Emery, Tom McNab and Professor Peter Wood.

6

The Woman Dieter

In this era, when inflation has assumed alarming proportions and the threat of nuclear war has become a serious danger, when violent crime is on the increase and unemployment a persistent social fact, 500 people are asked by the pollsters what they fear most in the world and 190 answer that their greatest fear is "getting fat."

—Kim Chernin
The Obsession

I suppose you really do believe that your happiness is consequent on your size? That an inch or two one way or the other would make you truly loved? Equating prettiness with sexuality, and sexuality with happiness? It is a very debased view of sexuality you take, Phyllis. It would be excusable in a 16-year-old—if my nose were a different shape, if my bosom were larger, if my freckles were gone, then the whole world would be different. But in a woman of your age it is vulgar.

—Fay Weldon
The Fat Woman's Joke

FAT IS SEEN AS WRONG

Fear of fat and desire to lose weight obsess women in our society. Slimness is associated with glamour, success and beauty. As the Duchess of Windsor said, "A woman can never be too rich, or too thin."

The image of the fat man retains an attraction, as an embodiment of power (Winston Churchill) or of joviality (Falstaff). But the image of the fat woman, the "earth mother," has been rejected. Fat women are penalized far more than fat men. Fat girls are less likely to gain college admission than thin girls, they are less likely to be given help of any kind, they are even more likely than the disabled to be rejected socially. And they cannot find fashionable clothes that fit them.

Fat is seen as wrong even by the very young. In 1978 three researchers from the University of Cincinnati College of Medicine presented a group of preschool children with two life-size rag dolls, identical except in one respect—and found that 91 percent of the children preferred the thin doll to the fat doll. And they also found that although the small number of overweight children in the group correctly perceived themselves as looking like the fat doll, they all preferred the thin doll.

In the same study the children were presented with line drawings of children of their own age, varying according to weight, sex and age: for example, a fat white girl, a fat black girl, a thin white boy. The children were asked to pick out which drawings they "especially liked" or "disliked" and those they thought were "weak," "happy," and so on.

All the children preferred the thin children. The investigators wrote: "There were three substantial trends: to see fat girls and thin boys as antisocial, to rate boys as more competent than girls, and to describe thin children as more competent than fat children." In other words, their peers mark out fat girls as inept and unattractive long before they have a chance to prove their talents and sociability at school.

After a study undertaken in 1963 the nutritionist Professor Jean Mayer, now President of Tufts University, stated:

When obese subjects demonstrate attitudes similar to those resulting from ethnic and racial prejudice, it is not far-fetched to say that obese persons may form a minority group suffering from prejudice and discrimination.

Women's fear of becoming fat, and their perennial dieting, spring from sources deeper than taste or fashion. In our society only thin is good.

A PERSONAL TALE

I became a devotee of the cult of slenderness when I was nineteen, in my first year at university. I expected great things from university. What I got—among other things—was my first experience of institutional cooking and communal eating. It was a shock.

In the first term, we had to eat breakfast in college. I was appalled, fascinated too, by the cornflakes, greasy fried eggs, mounds of baked beans and floppy white bread. However, I did what was expected of me, and dug in. And in a strange new world, for those first lonely few weeks, food was comforting. I felt sick and dull quite a lot of the time, but I had been brought up to eat up; mealtimes in my family were a recognized source of pleasure.

In eight weeks I gained 10 pounds. I was horrified. For the first time in my life I felt gross.

I came to loathe the smell of stewed cabbage and gravy, and began to associate the gray lukewarm meals with the girls who ate them. I shrank from the image I saw of hundreds of pasty faces wolfing down fodder. My fear, I now recognize, was of being swallowed up by the mass, of losing my own identity.

Eating punctuated every occasion. The cakes, the chocolate, the teas and biscuits, the late-night cocoa, the furtive and not-so-furtive candy bars, as essays were written or confidences swapped! We were lonely and unhappy girls, stuck out in remote and drafty buildings, eating as compensation, not for pleasure. I was disgusted and miserable. One day there was only one pair of trousers I could wear. I panicked. This was not, could not be me. I decided with compulsive urgency that I had to reject this environment.

I needed an image, an identity, that worked for me and was as distinct as possible from those around me. So I decided to get thin. Returning for the second term, I began my campaign. I still remember my first evening back. I announced that I "didn't want" dinner and went to bed early with a mug of hot milk, feeling excited, empty and nervous. I had been brought up to eat properly; this was a whole new experience.

I became good at calorie counting. Soon I knew the energy content of scores of foods by heart. Fruit, yogurt, crispbread and endless cottage cheese, salads; these became my eating routine. As often as not conversation revolved around food and slimming. I read dieting magazines. Proper sit-down meals made me nervous. Life was busy. I cycled everywhere, and I became addicted to the process of slimming. I swung from highs to lows; from feeling on top, beautiful, in control, to troughs of feeling depressed, weak, defeated. I came to associate the lows with "feeling fat," and forced myself back to ever fiercer self-denial.

After a few days' fasting I would go back to my mouse portions of cheese and crispbread, with "rewards" of chocolate. When I did go out to dinner, the next day was a day of penance. I loved being skinny. It was the mark of my self-control. I wore tight jeans and a navy sweater for nearly all my four university years to emphasize my streamlined image. And I was encouraged by other girls' remarks. "How thin you are!" they said. I heard envy and admiration.

I wasn't aware how thin I had become; I rarely weighed myself. When my jeans were tight, I felt fat: as long as I remained at size 10 I was happy. I'm five foot seven and a half; at that time I weighed 120 pounds, sometimes as little as 115 pounds. I suppose I approached the state of anorexia nervosa. But I did eat regularly, even if the quantities were tiny, and I did eat meals when avoiding them would have meant embarrassment or confrontation—at home, for instance. Nevertheless, over a period of six years I became very attached to my own habits, always preferring a snack to a meal—which also meant eating cake or a cookie, as well as fruit, rather than something substantial and cooked. My unexpressed fear was that if I ate normal meals regularly I would lose control of my body.

I realize now that I kept myself permanently undernourished. Looking back, my high times were memorable. But they were peaks rising from valleys of depression, listlessness and fatigue. I usually felt cold. My digestion was bad. I suffered from anxiety. I suppose I assumed that these malaises were the human condition, woman's condition, or my personal bad luck. It did not occur to me that dieting was making me ill. I thought that to be thin was to be healthy—by definition.

Later on in London, no longer living alone, I could not avoid meals. Gradually and with some pain, I began to recognize my fear of food as a neurosis. My obsession with a super-slim profile began to fade, but it took a long time to stop panicking as I put on weight, to stop assuming that I would be judged and rejected in terms of my weight, to stop putting an image before the needs, health and fitness of my body.

And I began to see, too, the irony of the obsession that so many women have with their weight today. It is taken for granted that to be attractive women must be slim. How remarkable that at a time when women have never been freer to express their opinions and exercise their rights, they are most bound to constrain the shape and weight of their bodies, by dieting.

FEAR OF FATNESS

The 1983 Royal College of Physicians' report on obesity cites a recent estimate that, at any one time, 65 percent of British women are trying to lose weight; and that of the 31 percent of the population who are regular users of one or more slimming products, most are women.

Statistics indicate the extent of dieting. They cannot convey the emotional involvement or the cost in terms of money, time, energy and pain. The 1982 report of the *Economist Intelligence Unit* on health products states that dieting

is no longer to be seen as a special activity separate from
normal eating. We have moved, the EIU report claims, "toward the concept of weight management as part of regular
personal health care." But for women, dieting is less a question of "weight management" or "health care" than it is a
way of life.

Clair Chapman is an actress with the Spare Tyre Theatre
Company, a British comedy cabaret group whose acts comment on the state of women and their bodies. Interviewed in
December 1981 she said: "I was put on a diet by my mother
when I was twelve. Dieting was an initiation to womanhood. I
thought women just had periods and dieted."

Indeed, many women have come to know the cycle of
dieting and relapse, pounds lost and pounds regained, as
intimately as they know their menstrual cycle. The discomfort of self-denial is followed by the guilt of eating again,
while the body gradually becomes more and more flabby, not
just in the mind, but in reality.

Katina Noble, another actress with Spare Tyre, said:

> I remember how humiliated I was when my boy-
> friend said I must get some weight off before we
> went on a holiday abroad. How desperate I felt, on
> going to a hypnotist and finding a money grabbing
> charlatan. After eight years of this I was just so
> neurotic. I went up and down between 8½ and 12
> stone, but I was just as suicidal at 9 stone 4 as I was
> at 11 stone 12. I went to such lengths to cover up!
> Making sure the upper arms weren't showing, never
> showing my bottom, not wearing trousers for six or
> seven years; I used to wear a skirt down to my
> ankles. My whole life was piles of clothes.

A turning point precipitates many women into the dieting
cycle. Very often this turning point is adolescence, fear of the
sudden curves, thighs and breasts of womanhood. Sometimes the crisis is pregnancy, when the body not only contains another being but also gains weight fast. Postnatal
depression compounds the alienation a mother may feel from
her own body, and she may throw herself into a diet which
fights her needs and those of her baby at just the time when,

if she is breast-feeding, she most needs proper and nourishing food.

Other women diet because of approaching middle age. Refusing to accept it, they try to stay slim as a way of proving that they are still young. For these women aging is to be feared, in a society that prefers the freshness of youth to the wisdom of years. So often in middle age women subject themselves to chronic undernutrition and lose their self-esteem.

Diet clubs report that 90 percent of their clientele are women. The readership of diet magazines is similar. *Slimming,* once published and edited by Audrey Eyton, author of *The F-Plan Diet,* has a circulation of 321,000.

Women's therapy centers have now been founded in London and New York. The center in London reports that a quarter of the calls it receives every week are about eating problems. One letter in the weekly magazine *TV Times* provoked a mailbag of 800, all from women asking for help with eating problems. Almost 90 percent of the patients of a special clinic for eating disorders set up in Cincinnati in 1977 are women, and all are extremely distressed by their apparent lack of control over eating behavior. In some cases the eating patterns they exhibit are quite deviant from those of the normal population, but often they are unremarkable, except for the tremendous guilt they engender.

Why do we see only slim women as beautiful? Why are anorexia nervosa and other eating disorders increasing? Why has dieting mania gone so far that the top "nonfiction" bestsellers are diet books, in the United States and now in Great Britain as well? Why are women so uncomfortable with their bodies?

THE WOMAN AS PROVIDER

Traditionally, women have been denied the power to shape and control their lives. But they have enjoyed sovereignty in two areas: food and nurture, and beauty and the body.

Food, feeding, feasting, eating, cultivation, harvest: these are all concepts rich in meaning and ritual. Notwithstanding our mechanized world of fast-food chains, and brightly packaged food crammed with chemicals, everything that food stands for retains its symbolic meaning much more than we may care to realize. To offer food is still a primary act of hospitality, acceptance and love. And the principal responsibility for feeding, as for all other forms of nurture, has always fallen to women. The first food of life comes naturally from the mother's own body.

It is the woman who shops, cooks, feeds her man and her children. It is her responsibility to make food wholesome and appetizing. Every day she provides for her family. Yet our culture teaches her to beware of feeding herself. Next to recipes for mouth-watering meals, magazines print the latest diet instructions. In one feature women are taught to create a miracle of meringue and cream; in the next to avoid the temptation of cream puffs.

Women are bred to this double-think. Many become good at it. Others become what are now termed "compulsive eaters": they eat neurotically, usually too much—sometimes too little—in response to signals that have little to do with real hunger or appetite.

Women who restrict themselves to 1000 to 1500 calories a day subject themselves to voluntary semistarvation. The diet ended, the woman is liable to fall on food with an intense and insatiable hunger that persists for a remarkably long time. This is why the dieter, ending the prisonlike sentence of the regime, so often celebrates with what may very well be the first of another series of binges.

Thus are the seeds sown for compulsive overeating: uncontrolled eating of entire gateaux, quarts of ice cream, shelves full of food by night as well as by day. The dieter is aware of what is happening, finds no way to stop and is full of despair.

THE NEW RELIGION

These cycles of denial and reward, starvation and gorging, are familiar to many seasoned dieters. In *Fat Is a Feminist Issue*, Susie Orbach says that American women spend $10 billion a year on weight-control methods. There are five chains of diet clubs in Great Britain, all thriving, and more in the United States. In the United Kingdom, Weight Watchers alone runs 14,000 groups where 45,000 people meet weekly. Late in 1982, *People* magazine reported on the Cambridge Diet, a soluble powder sold at mass rallies by 177,000 "counselors" throughout the United States who make $6 on every $20 can.

> One after another they rose to testify. "We are part of a fresh spring rain to wash clean the body of mankind," enthused one of the faithful. "He is Julius Caesar," wept a follower, referring to the leader. "He is everything! Isn't he gorgeous! Our leaders do love us! This is a magnificent church!"

Diet is taking on the forms of religion: churches, prophets, bishops, priests, confession, surrender, redemption, and communion celebrated not with bread and wine, the symbols of an age-old meal, but with chemicals. The dos and don'ts of the diet books are the new dogma, the lists of forbidden and allowed foods the new catechism; and the diet doctor replaces the priest and physician of the past as woman's guide to grace. When organized religion is absent, other rituals take its place. It is no accident that dieting is most widespread and diet doctors most powerful in those countries, mostly Protestant, where religion has lost its grip. And just as Christians are taught that their bodies are vessels of sin and that salvation is through faith, so dieters can come to believe that their struggles and their failures only prove the need constantly to discipline and punish the body.

THE GILDED CAGE

Women's second domain is beauty and the body. It has often been said that the ideals of female beauty, and the yearly changes in the fashion industry, are both functions of man's impulse to limit women's development. Beauty gives women a certain power over men; indeed, seduction can be a woman's prime weapon. But the battle is lost before she begins, for beauty takes much maintaining, and beauty, alone of the instruments of power, wanes with age.

Of the 1001 people whom *Which?* magazine interviewed for its *Way to Slim,* 58 percent of the women wanted to slim for cosmetic reasons, contrasted with only 19 percent of the men. The women who were dieting for their looks were also the least overweight. Rather than concerning themselves with their health and fitness and with encouraging an inner beauty, women have—certainly until very recently—been preoccupied with gilding their cages. They spend vast sums of money on cosmetics and clothes, on polishing, manipulating and pummeling their bodies.

In Great Britain alone, over 10 million images of women naked to the waist are printed every day in popular newspapers. The female body is everywhere—on billboards and magazine covers, in store-window displays selling liquor, car radios, windows, cheese, insurance and rust remover. As we wait for a train our eyes are forced to wander over bits of women displayed on posters—legs here, a torso there, a smile, a head of hair, the Lee bottom. The images and the fantasies that go with them say: "Use our product, look beautiful, and men will buy you chocolates and jewels, wine you and dine you, marry you and make you happy." Like the products her body is used to sell, woman becomes a commodity on the market. She is both bait and catch.

Advertisements also prompt everyone—men as well as women—to see female bodies as objects. Jo Spence, a photographer who collects images of women, has observed the fragmentation techniques used by advertising agencies. In Gina Newson's television film *Body Images,* made in 1981, she said:

> You get on one page a pair of lips, you turn over and there's a pair of legs; turn over and there are eyes; turn over and there's a face that's been hacked in half by the edge of the page. It turns the woman into a fetish. She's completely ripped out of time. A little bit of her comes to represent her, in the image.

It is hard for women to see themselves whole. Neither, very often, do men see women whole. "I'm an ass man." "I'm a tits man." "I go for legs." Less cheerfully, women also fix their attention on parts of their body. "My bottom is too big." "My nose is all wrong and my bosom is too small." "My problem is my lumpy thighs." Men and women both think of women's bodies as a collection of parts. Living in an age when defective parts of machines, and now defective organs inside the human body, are pulled out, thrown away and replaced, women feel a constant need to change the "defective" parts of their body.

THE SELF-HATRED SYNDROME

A woman is aware that her own body does not compare well with the bodies she sees on the posters. Many women come to hate their bodies, and with the help of doctors try to treat their "defective parts" as if they were machinery. In 1979, 300,000 American women had their breasts enlarged, usually with silicone implants; and every year between 15,000 and 20,000 American women have their breasts reduced in operations that frequently fail, leaving them disfigured. Barbarous methods of losing weight have now been devised. Bypass surgery to remove a portion of the intestine is usually followed by severe, prolonged and repulsive gut problems that can kill. Stapling, an operation that closes off the upper portion of the stomach with sterilized staples, is also dangerous, and the staples are liable to tear.

Jaw-wiring has been in the news recently. This is a procedure which requires a woman to live on a liquid diet for a year or more, with her jaws wired shut. Any woman put on this regime will of course lose weight, and after a while she will learn how to talk, after a fashion. The long-term "success" rate of jaw-wiring is not known, because it is a new technique. But a few cases followed up after the jaws have been unwired show massive and dramatic weight gain. The following report appeared in the British daily newspaper the *Sun* in January 1983:

> Hairdresser Lynne Oakley, who shed 10 stone in two years, has put most of it back on again—in two

months. The wires doctors put on her jaws to stop her eating snapped before Christmas—and so did her willpower. Lynne, 30, who tips the scales at 24 stone, said yesterday: "It happened at the worst time when everybody was eating and drinking." She was down to 15 stone when she abandoned her battle of the bulge. Now she's going to start again.

Most of the women who submit themselves to these procedures are grossly obese, to the point at which their lives are in danger; or their obesity prevents some other surgical operation. But some women who are not by any means obese have found doctors willing to carry out these procedures. What causes the self-hatred that drives women to these drastic measures? It is not merely because their bodies do not conform to current standards of attractiveness. A young girl in Gina Newson's film says:

> I remember hearing this poem once, by Leonard Cohen. He was writing about his mother. He said, "She viewed her whole body like a scar grown over some earlier perfection." And I knew what that meant as if I'd written it myself, I knew from my soul. There's some very nice "me" inside and it's just spoiled by the way I look. I feel so fat and ugly.

The girl was shown in silhouette; she could not bear to be seen. Gina Newson told me that she was normal size, even on the slender side, and was in no way ugly.

For women fatness means ugliness, and to be ugly is to be rejected, lonely, on the margins of society. And so, by an appalling association of ideas, some girls and women who are lonely and feel rejected come to believe that this is because they are ugly and fat, even when by any sensible standard they are no such thing. No wonder women go on diets. In dieting, women turn their energies in on themselves, and concentrate on the private safe world of their own body. Of course, when the diet fails, they feel let down. Dieting begins as a comforting occupation which avoids conflict and engagement with the world outside, and then becomes a new and inescapable ground on which battles are lost.

These wars start early. The young girl with anorexia nervosa uses her body both as an object of her own will and as her one means of self-expression. Abandoning interaction with her family and with the world, the anorexic girl holds tight to the only territory which she feels to be her own: her shrinking body. Some anorexics say they would rather die than give up this control. Some do die.

Although anorexia is defined as a disorder separate from dieting, many anorexics begin by dieting. However it may be triggered, anorexia nervosa is not a disease but a neurosis, a severe maladaptation with a background of circumstances which are common to all women. Cases of anorexia nervosa are increasing, and are no longer confined to middle-class adolescent girls.

In her classic work *Eating Disorders: Obesity, Anorexia Nervosa and the Person Within,* Professor Hilde Bruch outlines hundreds of case histories. Anorexics, she says, tend to be above average in intelligence, and speak lucidly about their feelings. One girl whom Professor Bruch was treating said: "This was something I could control. I know my body can take anything." Another, by contrast, was afraid of being strong: "Her ideal was to be weak, ethereal and thin, so that she could accept everybody's help without feeling guilty." For Sheila MacLeod, who has written of her own experience in *The Art of Starvation,* being plump suggested being fattened for the kill; alternatively, being swallowed up by family, school and university.

For some women, becoming thin is a bid for autonomy. The woman with developed pathological anorexia goes so far as to deny anyone access to her when offered food, or the comfort and love associated with food. This contrasts markedly with the dieter, who wants to fit in with society's standards. Anorexics lose any real perception of body size; they cannot see that they are becoming skeletal.

New eating disorders are now being identified. The latest to hit the headlines of the women's pages is bulimia. Bulimics have a normal body weight, which they maintain by vomiting, as often as two or three times a day. Some women use this means of controlling their weight for years. So too do some sportsmen who must keep their weight down—jockeys, for example. Bulimia, which is painful unless you have de-

veloped stomach muscles, eventually strips teeth of their
enamel and soaks the digestive system with acid. Vomiting to
avoid weight gain is a practice that the bulimic will keep
secret. In our society, it isolates her even more than the
taking of illegal drugs.

A single small announcement was placed in the British
edition of *Cosmopolitan* asking bulimic readers to complete
a questionnaire. Over 1000 replies were received. Over half
this number of women made themselves vomit at least daily;
about 70 percent were generally disturbed; 89 percent had
"profoundly disturbed attitudes to food and eating." Although most of the women felt they needed medical help,
only 30 percent had mentioned their habit to a doctor.
Bulimia is not often noticed, because sufferers usually eat
normally and have a normal weight, while the sense of shame
and disgust they feel keeps them underground. Magazine
articles in which women talk about having been anorexic are
quite common nowadays. But I have yet to read a piece about
a woman who says that she throws up and is proud of it.

WOMEN, FOOD AND SOCIETY

There is something wrong with a society that drives women
to diet constantly, to starve themselves beyond help, to void
their food, yet these things are commonplace in our society.

The condition of women preoccupied with their weight
is pitiable: they blame themselves, punish themselves, allow
themselves to be subjected to "aversion therapy" in which
they receive an electric shock when confronted with chocolate, join diet clubs in order to retrain all thoughts about food,
believe that their instincts to be nourished are bad.

For dieters the fear of food develops because diets do
not work and only increase the desire for food. No wonder
that so many women have "disordered" eating habits.

Priests and doctors have put the weight of their authority
on the side of body hatred. Within Christianity the spirit is at
war with the flesh and, since the Fall, it has been woman's
flesh that has tempted man into evil. The Virgin Mary, pure
and beautiful and often depicted as slim, is not an exception

and proves the rule—for, unlike any earthly mother, she is a virgin. In *The Second Sex,* Simone de Beauvoir writes:

> The flesh that is for the Christian the hostile *other,* is woman. In her, the Christian finds incarnated the temptations of the world, the flesh and the devil. All the fathers of the church insist on the idea that she led Adam to sin.

Christianity associates woman with the earth, with the old pre-Christian religions and so with the devil, whom Christians pictured as a perversion of the horned gods worshiped in Europe before Christianity. Women who understood the ways of the earth, knew the plants and herbs that would restore well-being, heal wounds and help in illness, were labeled witches and destroyed, and much of their knowledge with them.

In the Middle Ages and well beyond, church and state both enforced fear and suspicion of woman's body. "Get thee to a nunnery," Hamlet says to Ophelia, who goes mad. Othello eventually believes that Desdemona is lustful and murders her. Chastity belts, female circumcision, convents, chaperons were all means used to protect men against the supposed carnal impulses of women, and to protect women from themselves.

Rampant suspicion of women's sexuality lay behind many so-called "scientific" beliefs propounded by doctors in the nineteenth century. *The Journal of the American Medical Association* in 1894 recommended treating sexual desire at the menopause with hot douches of up to ten quarts daily and leeches to take fluid from the region of the uterus. The physician's conclusion sounds much like that of a modern diet doctor. "Such patients have so much lack of confidence in themselves, their physicians and their friends, that they have not the willpower to keep up a systematic course of treatment."

Writing in 1910, Havelock Ellis found that the belief, spread by doctors as scientific orthodoxy, that men and women breathed differently—men "abdominally" and women "thoracically"—stemmed from the fact that the women measured had crushed their stomachs with corsets.

In *The Unfashionable Human Body,* social historian Bernard Rudofsky says: "The physician, whose business it is to keep us in good working order, was then as reluctant to interfere with fashion's dictate as he is today."

Jane Fonda to her cost found that Rudofsky was right when, as a model and then as a film star, she not only dieted obsessively but, to force her weight down, took drugs for over ten years.

> No doctor ever told me of their side effects. No doctor ever took the time, or showed enough interest, to ask just how and why we were using these amphetamines. Nor did any doctor warn us that we could become addicted to them—as I did.

Today, food has replaced sex as the focus of women's self-disgust and guilt. It is fatness that leads to damnation: slimness through dieting is the salvation.

However, the futility of dieting fuels some women's sense of worthlessness. Others diet because they feel that as long as they are fat—in their own eyes—their life has not started, and that dieting will solve their problems. "When I am thin, then . . ."—I will be beautiful, or healthy, or lovable, or happy, or successful, or effective. The *Which? Way to Slim* gives sober counsel to its readers:

> Losing weight will not of itself guarantee that you will find a marriage partner or improve your relationship with the one you have. You should regard your slimming as a rational task which will result in weight loss—not as a magic solution to all your ills.

THE FRAGILE IDEAL

Has woman's flesh always been despised? By no means. The image of the Earth Mother has its origins in agriculture. It was women, there is little doubt, who first tilled the soil, planted, sowed and cultivated the earth, and gathered in the harvest. When settled communities began to be established, it was the women with flesh who were best protected against times of famine, and most likely to bear healthy children. Fertility symbols often depicted hugely fat women.

The connection between beauty and the promise of fecundity has been made for centuries in art. The paintings of Rubens and Rembrandt, and later of Courbet and Renoir, all celebrate the abundance of female flesh and a voluptuous sexuality.

In Europe, slenderness in women first became fashionable in the eighteenth century. In the Age of Enlightenment, the emerging middle classes had less fear of disease, plague and famine were no longer rampant, and the food supply was more assured. Man required a companion on his now extended journey through life.

The woman of leisure came to be associated with the finer things of life: with art and literature, taste and refinement. The wife of the peasant continued to be buxom; the wife of the gentleman was sensitive, her elegantly slender body betraying little sign of the basic functions of life, her soft white hands giving no sign of work, her delicate complexion unmarked by weather. That, at any rate, was the ideal.

As the concept of companionship implies, women were being raised from an entirely subordinate role to one of greater equality, one more "like men," and they began to aspire to the physique that went with the role. In her book *Fat and Thin,* medical historian Anne Scott Beller says:

> People tend to ape their betters, and women's aspirations to the unmodulated physiques of men express unvoiced, and until recently probably largely unconscious, judgments about the nature of male status and privilege compared with their own.

But the ladies of the eighteenth century, with their wit, charm and intelligence, posed a certain threat to men. The next century was to remedy that situation by developing the ideal female shape in another direction.

The nineteenth-cenutry lady was fragile and languorous, liable to fainting fits and to the vapors. Her vulnerability emphasized the strength, power and superiority of the man.

The pallor of a Dame aux Camélias was a sign of an all too delicate constitution. Consumption became chic. This ethereal creature did not so much diet as starve herself. She was too unworldly for such coarse matters as food. She took enemas and purgatives to maintain her tiny waist. Her tightly laced corsets made sure she could not digest food properly when she did eat. Her body weak and crushed, she often miscarried. That, at any rate, was the image to which so many Victorian women were expected to aspire, and their failure, as their bodies resisted their regimes, must have made them as guilty and ashamed as any female dieter today.

In *Illness as Metaphor,* Susan Sontag says:

> Twentieth-century women's fashions (with their cult of thinness) are the last stronghold of the metaphors associated with the romanticizing of TB in the late eighteenth and early nineteenth centuries.

INDEPENDENCE OR VULNERABILITY

Since the early 1960s—years in which the contraceptive pill has removed the risk of pregnancy from sex, and the women's movement has grown—dieting has engulfed the women of the West. In some respects the compulsion to diet is similar to the contrasting forces behind the ideals of slimness prevailing in the eighteenth and nineteenth centuries. Today, some women diet to assert their sexual freedom, seeing the sexually active body as lean, smooth and honed. Others, by contrast, diet to show an appealing vulnerability, seeing the slim, submissive body as soft and petted. These opposing ideals can resonate against each other, causing new confusions. An unpleasant recent example is the rise of the child model and movie star, the adolescent bodies of Brooke Shields and Jodie Foster becoming sex symbols in *Pretty Baby* and *Taxi Driver.* Ever since Twiggy's astounding success as a model in Great Britain and the United States, millions of women have half-starved themselves in futile attempts to achieve her figure.

Hilde Bruch comments:

It is impossible to assess the cost in serenity, relaxation and efficiency of this abnormal, overslim fashionable appearance. It produces serious psychological tensions to feel compelled to be thinner than one's natural make-up and style of living demand. I do not know how often people are aware of the emotional sacrifice of staying slim.

As time passes women very often find that unless they exercise, the only way they can stay slim is to submit to a state of perpetual semistarvation, in which they may also have to take drugs, and are quite likely to form disordered eating patterns. The consequence is depression, exhaustion and illness, and a reduced life expectancy. In these circumstances it is better to fail. Professor Bruch continues:

> There is a great deal of talk about the weakness and self indulgence of overweight people who eat "too much." Very little is said about the selfishness and self indulgence involved in a life which makes one's appearance the center of all values.

We all need a sense of control over ourselves and our lives. The language women dieters use to describe their fears is significant. "I mustn't let myself go." "I'm afraid of my fat taking me over." "My body's out of control." "I feel helpless when I gain weight." But the sad irony is that dieting itself alienates the body and produces the weakness, illness and flabbiness that the dieter most fears. Dieting is now the most widespread self-destructive activity known to woman.

Mastery is a male concept. The women most concerned to prove themselves the equal of men, in men's domains such as business and industry, are particularly likely to see pencil thinness as a sign of dynamism, of mind over matter, and a rigid armor typical of the male executive. The image is not that of an earthy siren—a Dorothy Lamour, Marilyn Monroe or Sophia Loren—but of heady adventuresses such as Bette Davis, Joan Crawford and Katharine Hepburn, mannish, independent and tough.

Other women, trying to reconcile their conflicting desires to be all things to all people—to be worker and wife, lover and mother, to work well in the office and at home, to satisfy colleagues, man and children—are liable to compensate for the lack of control they feel over their lives by retreating into the one area they think they can control: their bodies. Sadly, defeat in dieting is likely to be the most inevitable defeat of all.

The swings from self-denial to self-indulgence, from fasting to feasting—all of which may involve secret or furtive eating—reflect woman's oscillation between her conflicting roles. For the younger woman the pressure is more than ever to be thin. The Superwoman image cultivated by Helen Gurley Brown of *Cosmopolitan* and by Shirley Conran in Great Britain is an image of both femininity and independence: these women represent themselves as having it all ways. "If only I could look like that," other women think, go on another diet, and fail again—and again.

Self-doubt, anxiety, lack of confidence, confusion, self-destructiveness: these are emotions most women know all too well. Successful women too: "Will I be lovable if I'm strong and independent?" "Will my children hate me for having a career?" "If I choose to stay at home and care for my family will I regret it later?" Women's magazines are full of questions like these.

But finally, the realization is dawning that dieting is a lonely and frustrating business that usually fails; and that the rules of the calorie charts, the instructions of the diet doctors, the obedience and submission involved in dieting, the fragility and weakness that come with loss of weight, are all repulsive as well as futile.

As they turn away from spending their lives being told what to do, women should also turn away from the regulations and restrictions and, yes, the persecution of dieting regimes and diet doctors. Men are more and more discovering the value of their emotional selves. Women have the opportunity to discover the strength and power of their physical selves.

This does not mean opting for the Earth Mother image, which is just as limiting as the Slender Superwoman stereotype. But it is time to abandon the notion that a woman needs to be thin to be a real woman. It is time that this adolescent image is seen for what it is, and for women to find out what is the best shape and size for themselves as individuals. It is time, too, to abandon the costly and futile wars that women fight against their own bodies, to abandon the diet regimes that weaken them, depress them and eventually—ironically—make them fat.

It is time for women to get on the move.

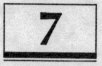

The Active Woman

It is vain to say human beings ought to be satisfied with tranquillity: they must have action, and they will make it if they cannot find it. Millions are condemned to a stiller fate than mine, and millions are in silent revolt against their lot. Women are supposed to be very calm generally; but women feel just as men feel; they need exercise for their faculties and a field for their efforts as much as their brothers do; they suffer from too rigid a constraint, too absolute a stagnation, precisely as men suffer.

—Charlotte Brontë
Jane Eyre

What is now called the nature of women is an eminently artificial thing, the result of forced repressing in some directions, unnatural stimulation in others. It may be asserted without scruple, that no other class of dependents have had their character so entirely distorted from its natural proportions.

—John Stuart Mill
The Subjection of Women

FINDING YOURSELF

For women exercise is a sure way of self-discovery and self-realization. Accustomed to see themselves, and be seen, as passive objects, many women find the effects of exercise a revelation. Interviewed in San Luis Obispo, California, for *Running* magazine, Alice Werbel spoke of her first running steps, age fifty-seven, and after her husband Ernie had retired:

> Your children are gone; you must get up and do something. We started to take long walks. We walked by the High School track and one day I said—why don't we run, just a quarter mile or so? Then one day, we got to run a mile.

That was in 1973. The first race Alice entered was the 10,000-meter run at the Senior Olympics held at Irvine. Her son had sent her a wool warm-up suit, and, knowing no better, she ran that race under the California summer sun wearing it. Nevertheless, her time of fifty-three minutes was a world record for women aged between fifty-five and sixty. In 1981 she held six world records, for distances between 800 meters and the one-hour run. In 1983, at the age of sixty-eight, she said, "I so often wish that people could understand that they had it within them. You feel sometimes that you shouldn't be out there training on the track; that you should be in a rocking chair."

At eight in the morning on Sunday, March 29, 1981, Sue Goggin, a forty-year-old mother of three, was at the gates of Greenwich Park to watch the start of the first London marathon. "Oh, what admiration I had for all those people, especially the old. If they can do it, so can I at forty," she wrote. She started to jog—finding at first that she couldn't run fast enough to catch the bus to work. Then she joined the London 1982/50 group, training for the second London marathon, on Sunday, May 9, 1982; she completed it in a time of four hours fifty-seven minutes. For her, running has given her a new freedom: "It is marvelous to shut the front door and leave all the hubbub and squabbles of three children behind—let Dad sort it out for a while, and feel the freedom of running with one's own thoughts."

Helen Johnston, a woman of twenty-eight, was part of the same London marathon team; she finished in four hours twenty-one minutes. For her, changed shape, not weight, was the main benefit of running:

> My weight has stayed much the same, although I eat more. Running makes me so hungry! A lot of women complain about flabby thighs. Mine used to be, but running has firmed them up—also backside. I just feel so healthy and fit!

CALM AND ZEST

Women report various benefits from exercise: sleep becomes deeper, period pains subside, they feel calmer and have more zest. Lucille Deane, another young member of the London marathon team, said:

> Physically I just felt more alive. I've always been rather a bad sleeper and suddenly I find, now, that I go out like a light. I feel that my body is using its food more efficiently. I don't feel hungry for at least an hour or two after a run. What I do eat I feel is being metabolized more efficiently now.

Some psychologists in the United States are discovering the effectiveness of exercise compared with conventional psychoanalytical methods in raising personal awareness and dealing with anxiety and depression. In her book *Women and Sports,* Janice Kaplan describes the work of Dyveke Spino, once a clinical psychologist and now an Olympic coach. Referring to the Greek ideal of the integration of mind, body and spirit, she says: "You can't deal with the mind and emotions unless you pay attention to sports and games." Using movement therapy and jogging and running, she encourages women to get in touch with an energy they were unaware they had: "Most women have a lot of self-doubt and built-in masochism. They don't really know themselves, and don't know how to go into the world and grab what they want."

A run can be just as effective a therapy for depression as a session on the couch. An American psychologist, interested in the benefits of jogging, gave one group of people conventional analysis for an hour, one by one, and took a second group out together for half an hour's run. The joggers showed more improvement in their general sense of confidence and well-being; and they saved a lot of money, too.

TO OWN ONE'S BODY

I began to jog, and then run, almost a decade after I became a student. For me the sensation of moving swiftly through the air unhampered by the usual layers of clothing, handbag and high heels was extraordinary. On my first runs, just of ten and then twenty minutes, I felt the flush of warmth through my body as my sluggish circulation started to work; afterward, skin tingling, lungs heaving, I felt the glow of physical exertion and, later, the beginning of real hunger. These sensations, I came to realize with a pang, are those of childhood. A long time before, and I didn't know when, I had put them aside, along with tree-climbing and make-believe.

Mobility is crucial to the growth process of children; it is the key to their sense of themselves in the world. We cannot know much about our bodies unless we move them; and children are constantly on the move, touching and exploring the space around them and their place within it. Neurologist Paul Schilder's work has shown him that when children stop moving, they stop learning. This has special significance for the overweight and the obese. Commenting on Schilder's work in her book *Eating Disorders,* Professor Hilde Bruch writes, "The inactivity so characteristic of obese people thus appears to be related to their often disturbed body concept."

She is suggesting that some people become obese in part because of inactivity and, moreover, that inactivity is sometimes pathological, springing from fear of the world and fear of learning.

In the first months of running I made several other discoveries. My skin gained a bloom and a glow. Quite soon as my body adapted, I stopped puffing and gasping. I felt that my lungs were expanding, learning a new rhythm of inhalation and exhalation which soothed me as I ran. Without getting bulky my muscles started to become smoother and more defined; and my hair grew thicker and glossier. I gained respect for my body, which I had so often distrusted and despised.

At school and university, words had been my means of expression; I avoided games at school, I am a poor and fearful swimmer, and I never learned to play tennis. Sport was something sporty people did, so I was rather embarrassed to discover that I loved the experience and the effects of running. The world of physical expression is not one in which you can be smarter or cleverer; words don't come into it. It became a new way of being for me which I found exciting, liberating and even a little dangerous and scary.

I had no intention—nor have I now—of running races, let alone marathons; for me, the purpose of running is health and well-being. So as one running companion pushed me to run faster and longer, I moaned and complained: I was convinced that I couldn't do it, that I didn't want to do it, that it was too much for me. He was unimpressed; and to my surprise and—I must admit—pleasure, I found I could do more!

I began to test my new body on runs of first two, then three, then four and a half miles. It no longer mattered that I thought my body was less than perfect, because I was enjoying my body rather than looking at it from the outside. For the first time since childhood, I had the sense of living inside my own body.

After a few months of running three or four times a week, I found I had a real sense of hunger. In the mornings I looked forward to my breakfast—whole grain cereal and yogurt and a pot of tea—but no longer needed to have lunch just because it was "lunchtime." I eat now only when I'm hungry. My appetite for food increased spontaneously, which at first worried me. But I now know that the active body needs a lot of whole, unprocessed cereals and vegetables. At the same time my appetite for meat, sweets, chocolate, alcohol and cigarettes decreased. I still eat cakes and have a drink from time to time, and the occasional cigarette; but I no longer treat myself to a dessert as a way of trying to calm some general sense of dissatisfaction.

GAINING WEIGHT—LOOKING SLIM

I put on weight: about 6 pounds. The old part of me was horrified! But I was pleased with my body, and people kept telling me how slim I was: the catch-all compliment which often really means "How well you look!" I recognized, and it was a shock, that the feelings I used to label as neurotic—anxiety, depression, listlessness, hopelessness—were at least in part caused by my years of malnourishment and undernourishment. Angst is romantic, semi-starvation is not.

I started to enjoy listening to my body. For a while a series of malaises and infections made me feel as if running were in some way literally jogging poisons in my body to the surface. Whatever their cause, these illnesses ceased. Yoga classes, which I had previously put off when I believed I had something "better to do," became top priority; a couple of hours of stretching in a gym or an hour of running was never time wasted or lost, and gave me more energy and zest for my work. And I slept better.

When I started to exercise in the open air it was not just the exhilaration of movement that spurred me on, but also the forgotten joy of being in physical contact with nature. I had not realized just how much time I spent looking at the world through screens: windows; books, television, film; coats, hats, mufflers.

Running free, with minimum clothing, I got to know the world of Kensington Gardens and Hyde Park. I felt the different textures underfoot; tarmac, gravel, grass firm and muddy, snow. I watched the park grow as spring became summer, in different light and different weather. Wind and rain were simply that—cold and wet against the skin, bracing, not something to huddle away from. I felt the seasons change as shoots appeared; leaves emerged emerald-green, became darker in summer, then brown and gold in the autumn. I vividly enjoyed my new experience, as I passed by and came to know the people with their dogs, other runners whose route was clockwise, the tramp whose territory is a particular bench by the Royal Garden Hotel, the old lady forever painting the ornamental garden by Kensington Palace, from the east side of the vine arbor.

Exercising the body is a positive discipline, in contrast with the negative discipline of dieting. Any normal person longs for a diet to end. But once the body has become accustomed to exercise, a run, a dance session, a yoga class is something to look forward to: a freedom, not a restriction.

It all sounds simple and inviting. As Alice Werbel found, it is just a matter of acting like a child again—getting up and running, or swimming, or dancing, for fun. But for women there are more complex issues involved in exercise; Helen Johnston experienced one.

She found that many men need to believe that women are passive creatures, objects of admiration but not active, energetic and strong. She was the victim not only of verbal and sexual aggression from men as she passed by on the run, but also of threatened physical aggression.

> Most scary are the curb crawlers. I have nightmares of being dragged into the car. Then there are the pedestrians. The men are the most threatening and the most crude. All this upsets me, makes me angry, and sometimes I have honestly been very frightened.

When she started to run, Helen did not know how to handle this kind of bad experience. But once her body was in training she no longer cringed; she spoke out, and was able to answer the men back.

And there are other issues: taboos, self-doubt, family, social demands, prejudice, inhibitions, prohibitions.

LOSING AND WINNING

Again and again girls and women are prevented from participating in sports regarded as men's domain. In Great Britain, the Equal Opportunities Commission championed the case of Theresa Bennett, whom the Football Association had prohibited from playing in an under-twelve league. She won her case, but lost it on appeal. Evidence was put forward on Theresa's behalf that she was prepubertal and a "guided missile in football boots." Lord Denning set these pleas aside and refused further appeals, finally saying, "We don't inquire about the age of ladies."

Elizabeth Ferris, a doctor specializing in sports medicine, won the bronze medal for diving in the Rome Olympics in 1960. At school her headmistress had her examined by a cardiologist on the grounds that so much training must be bad for a girl's heart. A less determined girl would have been discouraged. Kathrine Switzer is public relations director of Avon Products, Inc., responsible for Avon's involvement in women's running. In 1967 she entered the Boston Marathon, purportedly an "open" event, as "K. Switzer," knowing that race officials would otherwise cancel her entry. As it happened, it took a hefty shoulder-charge from her boyfriend to prevent a race marshal from manhandling her out of the race, which she completed.

And it was not so long ago that award-winning football writer Brian Glanville of the *Sunday Times* made it clear that in his view sports were all right for women as long as they didn't get too competitive; "There is no reason why a woman should not indulge in any kind of sport she wishes." (It's difficult to imagine a writer saying: "There is no reason why a man should not indulge in any kind of sport he wishes.") Glanville goes on:

> A girl who goes out to run, swim, or play tennis for the joy of it is still being a girl. But a girl who slogs away all winter in a gymnasium lifting weights so she can beat other girls in the summer is behaving like an imitation man.

Winning is all right for boys. But a girl who wants to win—or even to exert herself to her utmost—is somehow unseemly. Rejecting a proposal that a woman's 3000-meter race should be included in the 1980 Games, the International Olympic Committee said that it was "a little too strenuous."

No wonder that a recent survey in Great Britain showed that only 40 percent of girls play any sports outside school. The boys had been encouraged; the girls had been discouraged.

COMPETING—AGAINST THE WILL OF MEN

The Olympic Games are supposed to be the summit of athletic ability and the manifestation of the true spirit of sport, where to win is not so glorious as to take part. But Baron Pierre de Coubertin, founder of the modern Olympic movement, fought successfully to keep women out of the Games. In the early years of this century, women's track and field events were organized separately from the Olympics. The first women's international meeting took place in Monte Carlo in 1921; over a hundred women from five countries took part. The next year it was decided to form a Women's World Olympics, but after pressure from Olympic Games officials the name was changed to the Women's World Games. These were held in 1922 in Paris, and 300 competitors from seven countries participated. Track events such as the 400 and 1500 meters were reduced to 300 and 1000 meters. For the second Women's World Games in 1926, in Sweden, ten countries were represented in thirteen events. In his book *Catching Up the Men,* Ken Dyer observed that at this point women's athletics "had grown from almost nothing to a major force on the sporting scene, with a program almost as varied as men's and approaching theirs in level of participant support." Only then was the perennial request that women be allowed to compete in the Olympic Games grudgingly accepted, for the 1928 Games. There were two conditions: women were admitted only provisionally and were confined to five events.

The all-male Olympic Committee thus effectively restricted what was becoming a flourishing and vigorous development. In the 1928 Games, held in Amsterdam, the 800-meter world record for women was broken by Lina Radke. As she and other competitors crossed the line, they collapsed from exhaustion. This precipitated a ban on all women's track races except the 100 meters, and thereafter the addition of each women's track event had to be fought for. The 800-meter track event did not reappear until 1960, the year in which Elizabeth Ferris competed as a diver. Addressing a congress on women and sport twenty years later, Dr. Ferris said:

> Even in 1960 only 600 of the 5,000 odd competitors were women, and they only competed in 6 of the 17 sports. We women, inside our very separate compound in the Olympic village, were savagely protected by patrolling guards who paced, panther-like, up and down outside a wire fence that was so high that not even the gold medalist in the pole-vault could have got over it.

The women's 200-meter race was added in 1948, the 400 meters in 1964 and the 1500 meters in 1972.

The hardest struggle for women in the Olympics has been to gain acceptance for long-distance running events. It was only in 1984 that the 3000 meters and the marathon were included. The absurdity of these delays is emphasized by the fact that it is in the endurance events that women's achievements are the greatest. Ann Sayer not long ago took the all-comer's record for the 840-mile Lands End to John O'Groats walk, beating the previous record set by a man. (Asked how she managed to finish in thirteen days, she said that she could take only two weeks off from work and had to be in the office the next day.) The American Penny Lee Dean is a holder of the England-to-France cross-Channel swimming record and Canadian Cynthia Nicholas of the two-way cross-Channel record. In 1980, Naomi James held the solo around-the-world sailing record. In long-distance endurance events women have less upper-body strength than men but compensate with comparable leg strength. And there is good evidence that in long-distance events women can regulate their body temperature better than men, and also that they use body fat as fuel more efficiently.

Avery Brundage, president of the International Olympics Committee from 1952 to 1972, always made it clear that he, like any good Victorian, thought women should be ladies. He once said, "I am fed up to the ears with women as track and field competitors. As swimmers and divers girls are beautiful and adroit as they are ineffective and unpleasing on the track."

In all professional sports, prizes for women professionals are far lower than those for men. But when they persevere and endure the training that makes champions, women are told they are "unfeminine." The great long-distance running coach Percy Cerutty had this to say: "Who wants straight-legged, narrow-hipped, big-shouldered, powerful women, aggressive and ferocious in physique and attitude?" Clearly such a woman would be more than Percy could handle!

Common sense suggests that in certain respects women have powers of endurance superior to those of men: women's bodies are built to bear children. Miki Gorman was the first woman home in the Boston marathons of 1974 and 1977, and in between had her first baby at the age of forty. "Compared with having a baby, a marathon is easy," she said. And during the 1970s, while the men's world record for the marathon remained at the 2.08.33 set by Derek Clayton, the women's world record was broken sixteen times, falling from 3.02.53 to 2.27.33. (In 1985 the men's record was still more than 2.08. Joan Benoit has lowered the women's record to 2.22.42.)

Why, then, did it take until the 1984 Games for the women's marathon to be accepted as an Olympic event? Elizabeth Ferris asked this question of a woman associate of the International Olympic Committee before the 1980 Moscow Games, at a time when thousands of women were competing in long-distance races. The reason given, said Dr. Ferris, was:

> She had seen a woman cross-country skier vomit at the end of a race, and this had offended her dreadfully. No woman, in her opinion, should be so exposed and vulnerable—it was against all her deeply

embedded views about what it means to be a woman.

EXERCISE AND "BEING A WOMAN"

It's not only the women athletes who have a hard time. We adapt to the roles expected of us very early in life. Little children playing at mommies and daddies will act out the mother at home, washing up, cooking, looking after the family; the father at the office being important, playing softball with his buddies on the weekend. Many television advertisements are versions of this game. No manufacturer ever sold a box of detergent by showing the man of the house exclaiming with wonder at the whiteness of his wife's shorts as he fishes them out of the washer. Men are meant to be strong and independent; women are meant to be gentle and dependent: we are all taught that. As they grow up, girls are encouraged to be more sedentary than boys. The very word "tomboy" used, affectionately or not, of a girl nearing puberty speaks worlds. A woman playing serious strenuous sport is as threatening as is a top woman executive; both women and men view such a woman as a challenge to the conventions of manliness and womanliness by which we live and limit our lives.

From time to time newspapers publish a story that women runners are liable to suffer from amenorrhoea (that is to say, their periods stop). Horror! The implication is that the athletic woman has lost her fundamental womanliness. Tales of tall high-jumpers and bulky hurdlers, usually from behind the Iron Curtain, who turn out by some criteria to be male, not female, also tie into this message: on the one hand, too much exercise is liable to render a woman neuter; on the other hand, some women athletes are men anyway.

Amenorrhoea is a common condition, as often as not caused by stress. It is perfectly true that periods are likely to stop or become irregular in a woman who trains very hard, running more than fifty to sixty miles a week, particularly if she is thin. The condition may be reversed by taking vitamin C and iron tablets, which are in any case advisable if she eats any amount of junk food and processed sugars. But there is no evidence that amenorrhoea induced by very heavy training continues after the training has eased off. Characteristically, though, the suggestion behind the newspaper stories is: don't jog, or you may not be able to have babies. This is nonsense. Exercise does not turn women into men, and it does not turn women neuter.

After starting to jog, I spent time worrying that I would develop bulging muscles—just like a man. Again, it is true that some female field athletes and body-builders develop musculature like that of men, but only if they take anabolic steroids—illegal drugs that contain male growth hormones. Without drugs, not even women weight-lifters develop bulging muscles. I had allowed myself to be inhibited by a myth; I did not do what was obvious—look at the women athletes to be seen any week on television.

WOMEN ARE CATCHING UP

Men's attitudes toward women in sports have been too easily accepted by women themselves. In the United States this attitude began to change dramatically in the 1970s. The staggering increase in interest in the long-distance running triggered by Frank Shorter's Olympic marathon win in 1972 disguised an even more extraordinary commitment from women.

In 1974 the ninth-place woman in the New York Marathon recorded five hours eighteen minutes. In 1983 the ninth woman recorded two hours twenty-eight minutes; and the women's field for the 1984 race, run on October 28, 1984, included 3,515 women. Women are beginning to catch up.

The movement for fitness through sport is also becoming a movement for health through exercise. Early in 1982, co-author Geoffrey Cannon invited people with no previous experience of running to train for five months with the goal of completing the two-and-a-half-mile *Sunday Times* National Fun Run. (This Fun Runner '82 project is described in Chapter 5, "More Air! More Air!") *Running* magazine, which carried Geoffrey Cannon's invitation for the Fun Runner '82 project, has a readership of 93 percent men to 7 percent women. Yet more than half of the 130 replies were from women. One said: "I desperately want to feel fit, healthy and mentally liberated from my two very adorable but demanding children. I would also very much welcome a challenge of this kind. Please be my savior!" Another replied simply: "My ambition is to become fit and healthy."

After three months of jogging, thirty-eight Fun Runners were asked if regular exercise had affected their mood: were they more, or less, anxious or depressed, from time to time? This question affected the women very much more than the men. Of the thirty-eight, twenty-one said that regular exercise had definitely improved their state of mind. How much difference? This is how they replied:

Bad mood, anxiety, depression	April	July
Every day	—	—
Most days	8	—
Most weeks	5	3
Occasionally	8	10
Hardly ever/Never	—	8

In July, one Fun Runner decided that she would stop seeing the psychiatrist who had been treating her for some time—simply because she felt fine.

The good effects of fresh whole food and of exercise are simple, and yet so often they are profound. The astonishing rise in the numbers of women who are physically active has been triggered not just by the urge to get fit, stave off heart attacks and middle-age spread, or cure depression—although these are good reasons. In my mind, it is also generated by the desire to rediscover the simple joy of feeling fully alive. The upsurge of running and dance is an appropriate reaction to our otherwise automated and sedentary lives.

"Energy is the power that drives every human being. It is not lost in exercise but maintained by it," said Germaine Greer in *The Female Eunuch*. Ten years later, Jane Fonda put Germaine Greer's thoughts into action, and the feeling of a new generation of women into words, in her *Workout Book*, saying:

I do not claim that a strong, healthy woman is automatically going to be a progressive, decent sort of person. Obviously other factors are involved in that. But I am sure that one's innate intelligence and instinct for good can be enhanced through fitness.

Watching others transform their lives through exercise, women sometimes say, or think, "It must be too late for me." The slinky goddess on television putting aerobics classes through their paces can be a discouraging sight. But even at the highest levels of achievement women are discovering that age is not a barrier to performance. Joyce Smith holds the British women's marathon record and was seen on television by millions, finishing ahead of the other women runners in the London marathon in 1981 and again in 1982—when she was forty-four years old. Beryl Burton, the long-distance cycling champion, continued to challenge male rivals well into her forties. Mary Peters won the Olympic Pentathlon in Munich when she was thirty-three. Miki Gorman continues to set world and American records for her age in the marathon. And for an older generation, the example of Alice Werbel, who started to jog when she was fifty-seven, can be an inspiration.

The time when her children grow up and leave home can be the time of a woman's life when she can use her experience and resourcefulness to discover a new taste for adventure, with an energy and steadfastness that many a young woman may envy.

THE BEAUTY OF STRENGTH

Exercise sheds fat and adds lean tissue, including muscle, to a woman's body. In action, the body of a woman who takes regular exercise is clearly toned; the shape of her muscle is unobtrusive, but it shows. Exercise creates strength, and many men other than Percy Cerutty are made to feel nervous by women who gain physical strength. But as women find just how good they feel about themselves after exercise, they are discovering a new inner beauty which isn't painted on.

Ken Kyer cites an interview with Anna Thornhill, an artist who is also a long-distance runner. She said:

> I don't worry about fitting in a fashion-type image anymore. After running a marathon and then a 7-mile race the next day and feeling no pains at all, I looked in the mirror and said, "Body, you're okay. You're doing your job."

And Ms. Thornhill also referred to another issue that women face. What will my man think of the way I look?

> My husband doesn't want me to become too thin, but I no longer want to surrender to someone else's view of sexuality; for me, functionalism and sexuality are fused. My sexuality isn't affected by the way I look anymore, but by how I feel: healthy, confident and functional.

Women, and men too, are learning that a notion of beauty as weakness and unhealthy softness is not a notion of beauty worth holding; that the firmness of the body and the inner glow that come with exercise are more attractive and lasting.

Some women are put off exercise because they half believe it will make them less of a woman. Others are afraid to exercise in public, either in a dance studio or in the open air, because they are only too well aware that they don't have the body beautiful of women in advertisements. Indeed, many women are afraid to show their bodies in private; sexual prudery often has little to do with morals, much more to do with fear of what the other person will think. Privately, women often hug thoughts that they are ugly or clumsy, even deformed.

Having summoned up courage to join in a jogging group or an exercise class, a woman may discover her first sense of freedom when she realizes that nobody looks like the women in the advertisements or the fashion magazines. Most models are made up and lit and photographed from special angles, to achieve an ideal effect which is not real. Stereotypes created by the camera, just as much as by the painter, do not exist in the flesh: meet a woman who is a model, and as likely as not her most attractive feature will be one regarded as a fault by fashion and so hidden in her pictures.

An exercise class gives a woman a chance to face her fantasies, including her own horrid fears about her own body, and realize that everybody looks different and that beauty is in the difference, not the similarities.

LOOKING GOOD—BEING YOURSELF

The second freedom for the woman who, at whatever age, starts to exercise regularly is that some of the features she dislikes and tries to disguise—dull complexion, flabby flesh, lumpy thighs—are liable to change, sometimes quite quickly, sometimes gradually. She begins to discover the natural shape of her body, a shape which, with exercise, she will begin to appreciate in new ways.

Physical exercise is not a panacea. It is hard work, and that is why the sense of well-being that comes from exercise is lasting: it is earned. People now are moving away from the idea of beauty that implies passivity, an idea that is a hangover from Victorian days. Slimness which depends on makeup, pills and diets has nothing to do with fitness or with health. As they enjoy the inner glow that comes from exercise, women today are contradicting the notion that beauty is only skin-deep. Diets treat the body as alien, as an enemy of the mind. Exercise treats the body as integral to us, as bound up with the mind and the spirit. After three months of jogging, Kathleen Herold, a thirty-eight-year-old member of the Fun Runner '82 group, wrote:

> If I don't run every day my body lets me know that something is missing. I have lost weight, my blood pressure is down, and my resting heart rate has lowered. Physically I am in better shape than I was 20 years ago; now I can run over two miles a day.

And Brenda Green, aged fifty-two:

> If I'm driving the car and see a runner I'm tempted to stop and join in—and I'm so pleased to see more

females running nowadays. I've now lost 10 pounds and big Sunday lunches are a thing of the past. I feel terrific: full of energy and confidence. I wish I had done all this years ago.

And the most engaging comment, in one of the newsletters the Fun Runners circulated to each other, came from Diana, the typist:

I used to enjoy typing and I thought it was good exercise. At least I had fit fingers! But I have spent the last half hour typing about other people's running and thinking how much I would rather be out running than in typing. So I'm going to turn the typewriter off now and get my running shoes out!

As we have seen, the Cattell 16 Personality Factor Questionnaire showed that at the end of the project the Fun Runners had become more self-confident; more understanding of the needs and problems of others; less apprehensive; better-mannered and less aggressive; and more relaxed and composed. Dr. Barrie Gunter was especially interested to note what had happened to the women:

I believe that improved aerobic capacity can bring with it a feeling of well-being for the relatively unfit person—especially when he or she compares the way they feel now with how they felt just a few weeks or months before.

Gunter emphasized that the most substantial shifts in personality occurred among women; for, according to his assessments, they started the project less self-assured, more tense and less emotionally stable than the men.

Given the pressure put on women right from the start of their lives to shrink away from their physical selves, these findings were hardly surprising. Wilhelm Reich has said: "Every disturbance of the ability fully to experience one's own body damages self-confidence as well as the unity of the bodily feeling. At the same time it creates the need for compensation."

The compensation women are accustomed to is a world where chocolates and flowers and jewels are advertised as signs of love; where glossy magazines encourage fantasies of exotic places and exotic men; where less glossy magazines encourage daydreams of romantic passion. These treats are substitutes for creating our own drama, activity, and excitement. Life is, should be, something we feel physically and experience through our bodies.

And this is what women are now finding out for themselves. In October 1982 I attended a conference called "The Exercise Boom" held by Pineapple Dance Studios in London. Women of all ages from eighteen to over seventy came from all over Britain to take part. Ex-model Jackie Genova and former Olympic athlete Cindy Golbert hold aerobic classes for hundreds of women at a time, in London. Jane Fonda's admirable *Workout Book* has been in the British best-seller lists for over a year and was on the American lists for almost two. New magazines aimed mainly at women who want to be healthy and fit—*Fit, Self*—and for men and women—*American Health*—have been launched in the United States. *Workout, Fitness,* and *New Health* have been launched in Britain. Early in 1983, *Running* magazine asked for applications from women, to train for the Avon women-only ten-mile race now held every October at Copthall Stadium in north London. The response, for a magazine 93 percent of whose readers are men, was awe-inspiring: 839 women wrote in. The mass-circulation magazine *Woman's Own* sponsored a series of ten-kilometer races for women only up and down Britain in September 1984. Led by Kathrine Switzer, Avon now sponsors ten-, fifteen- and twenty-kilometer races throughout the United States, for women only.

Aerobics, dance exercise, jazz exercise—these are not fads confined to the middle classes of London and New York. They are, all together, a new movement springing from and drawing encouragement from other and older disciplines.

A NEW HARMONY

Thérèse Bertherat is a French body therapist who doubts the value of exercise that amounts to drilling the body. She believes that those aerobic dance classes that are run by a woman who sounds like a shrill sergeant-major will only confirm a woman's fears that her body is inadequate. In her book *The Body Has Its Reasons,* Madame Bertherat writes:

> It is possible for you to find the keys to your body again, to find your proper vitality, health and autonomy. But how? Certainly not by regarding your body as a necessarily defective machine that encumbers you, as a machine made up of isolated parts, each of which must be entrusted to a specialist whose authority and verdict you blindly accept.

Yoga encourages us to listen to what our bodies can tell us. So do other disciplines from the East, such as aikido and tai chi, and some forms of movement therapy developed in the West, including bioenergetics and the Alexander Technique. Some women prefer vigorous, even exhausting exercise; the temperament of others will lead them into a quieter means to the same end. My friend, Barbara Dale, who runs the Body Workshop in London, teaches exercise based on the Mensendieck method. She uses toning and stretching as "active meditation" and combines them with the aerobic exercise that the body needs. She told me:

> I'm very aware that everything is reflected in your body. During the last 100 years we've come to realize that the mind is a tape of everything that's happened to you. People still don't realize that the body is the very same tape.

The aches and illnesses we suffer, the odd ways we have of sitting, standing, walking, are all part of our personal maps, from which, if we are attentive, we can learn more about ourselves. As I kept on running, I also learned something that previously I would have dismissed as silly and perverse. I learned that discomfort and even pain can be valuable experiences that show what the body can bear; and I enjoyed exploring my limits, and finding that they expanded. Exercise that one week would be uncomfortable, even painful, became easier the next, and so I wanted to try harder. How can we know who we are unless we try to extend our limits? How can we learn about ourselves without exploring?

It is believed that the left hemisphere of the brain governs our reason and the right our intuition; and that we in the West have allowed ourselves to be dominated by the left half of our brain. All acts of creation require intuition to interplay with reason, and genius is always inspired by guesses that have nothing to do with logic. The free flow of energy that results from exercise seems to come from our intuitive, even psychic side, and the sense of well-being that invariably follows vigorous exercise may very well derive from a harmony between our two sides.

For women—and men—whose lives are packed with work, stress, decisions and conflict, exercise may very well be the balancing agent.

Women are brought up to feed and care for others, to give their time, energy and love to supporting the activity of husband, children or boss. Many women feel uneasy, even guilty, at the idea of taking time to look after and nourish themselves. But just as no plant thrives without watering, no body flourishes without tender loving care. Women who take time each day to enjoy themselves in exercise and other forms of play are less prone to self-destructive feelings of resentment and helplessness. People cannot fully love others unless they have self-esteem. Many women, busy with home and children, neglect themselves, not realizing that a self-forgetful attitude breeds indifference and even contempt in others. No one ever thanked a wife or mother for saying, "I did it all for you."

SELF-NOURISHMENT

It takes some courage for a woman to give herself time for self-nourishment. Any woman accustomed to dieting will at first resist the idea that good health and a reliable and lasting sense of well-being come from balance between our two fuels, food and air, and from plenty of both. It is hard to appreciate, at first, that the foods most often condemned by diet books—bread, potatoes, root vegetables, cereals and pastas—are indeed the staff of life. New discoveries involve giving up old beliefs, and a woman who has spent five or twenty-five years going from diet to diet will not find it easy to accept the notion that her dieting was misspent time.

The self-nurturing and self-assertion involved in exercise go beyond good health. As they grow up, girls are so often discouraged from being competitive and many women deny that they are competitive because they have been taught to feel that in any of life's races they will fail. Exercise encourages a sense of success; a woman does not have to be first in a sport; she can achieve the physical goals she sets herself, and even outdo them. This self-realization will dissolve the jealousies and frustrations that women so often come to believe are part of everyday life.

As most women have found out for themselves, diets simply do not work. But millions of women, although they know that diets do not work for them, still believe that they are at fault, that they are weak, inadequate or greedy. This book is offered as a new freedom for all these women. Diets do not work: and it is their fault, not yours.

Through exercise and good food women can become fit, healthy, confident and full of energy, and can gain a new self-respect and control over themselves and their lives. By learning to love themselves, women will be able to love others better. By enjoying more of the good things in life, women can understand and discover themselves as whole people, strong, able, active and in harmony with men.

8

All You Need
to Know

It seems to me that we are still awfully ignorant of some basic biological knowledge regarding the nutritive value of food and its additives, its effect on the physiological activities of the gut, and the general metabolic consequences of this action.

—Sir Ernst Chain
*Food Technology in the 1980s,
Address to the Royal Society*

How we need that unity today, that glowing oneness of body, mind and spirit! More than ever, now that the modern era of careless indolence and gluttony is so clearly ending, we need the tingling aliveness of every limb, the connectedness with nature and other people that only a full appreciation of embodiment can bring.

—George Leonard
The Ultimate Athlete

The thesis of this book can be summed up in thirty points. The first ten summarize the effect of dieting on the human body.

1. Diet books assume that the body works at a set speed; that some people have a fast metabolic rate, others a slow one, but that the basic rate for each individual remains the same. All the sums in diet books that tell dieters how many calories to consume are based on this assumption. It is wrong. Metabolic rate is not static; it is dynamic.

2. Whatever the "thesis" of diet books, they all state or imply that most if not all weight lost on a diet is fat. This is not true. The initial big weight loss during a diet is of water, and of glycogen, a form of glucose stored together with water in the liver and the muscles. Glycogen is the body's immediately available source of energy, and is the fuel for the brain.

3. Weight lost on a prolonged diet is lean tissue from vital organs and muscles, as well as fat. The more severe the diet, the greater the proportion of lean tissue lost. Metabolic rate slows dramatically during a diet because much of the weight lost is tissue which, unlike fat, is designed to be metabolically active. Hence the slowing down of weight loss, as the diet continues.

4. The body of a person on a crash diet reacts as if to starvation; the body of a person on a prolonged diet reacts as if to famine. In each case the body will shed active tissue that consumes a lot of energy and as far as possible will protect the relatively inactive tissue which it is vital to store in times of starvation or famine. This inactive tissue is, of course, fat.

5. The human body is more complex than that of any other creature and continually adapts to circumstances. The body of an active person will adapt to protect and develop muscle that is constantly used. The body of a sedentary person loses muscle as life goes on. The body of a sedentary dieter will tend to shed muscle because it is little used.

6. Glycogen is essential to the functioning of the body and the brain. Loss of glycogen triggers sensations of intense hunger, even if the stomach is full of food. When a diet is ended the body will replace its glycogen store, and water. But the body of a sedentary dieter will tend not to replace all the metabolically active tissue that has been lost on the diet.

7. Constant dieting trains the body to endure diets. It does this by a process of shedding some lean tissue and replacing it with the fat needed at times of starvation and famine. Fat is itself a source of energy and needs less fuel than the vital organs. So the metabolic rate of the dieter tends to drop from one diet to the next; the body needs less and less food.

8. Loss of glycogen results in listlessness, depression and irritability. Loss of lean tissue, including muscle, diminishes the need for energy from oxygen in the air, as well as for energy from food, and the body comes into energy balance at a lower and lower level. Constant dieting makes a person feeble and torpid. This is a cumulative process.

9. Because a low metabolic rate often results from being fat, a fat person may "eat like a bird" and get fatter. On the other hand, a lean person may "eat like a horse" and stay lean, because of a high metabolic rate. Women need and use less energy than men; and a light yet fat middle-aged woman who diets regularly can gain weight even on a semistarvation diet.

10. Dieting slows the body down and creates the conditions for gaining fat. Gradually, after one diet has ended, dieters get fatter and fatter on less and less food. Fat weighs less than lean tissue, and it is perfectly possible to lose weight as a result of accumulative diets and nonetheless gain a greater volume, as well as proportion, of fat to lean tissue.

This is why dieting makes you fat. The next ten points summarize why up to half the population of Western countries tend to get fat, with or without dieting.

11. Diet books imply that the basic requirement of the body is energy from food. This is wrong. The body can and does adapt to very different levels of energy balance. The body's basic requirement from food is not for quantity but for quality. Above all, what the body needs is nourishment. What is wrong with the food we eat is not its quantity but its lack of quality.

12. Foods lose nourishment when processed. People in Western countries now eat more processed, "refined" sugars than any other item of food. Processed sugars are dead, or empty, energy. They supply calories but no protein, essential fats, fiber, vitamins or minerals. "Junk" foods supply calories but little or no nourishment. Processed sugars are the chief junk food.

13. Deficiency diseases are caused by a gross lack of nutrients. These diseases have mild forms that are difficult to diagnose and that may produce depression, exhaustion, swings of mood, anxiety, period pains, sleeplessness, irritability or irrational or destructive behavior. One prime cause of such malaise, almost universal in Western countries, is junk food.

14. The body will always defend itself against the threat of illness. The body of a sedentary person who eats an average amount of processed foods and sugar will continue to signal hunger until enough nourishing food has been eaten. The only way for such a person to get enough nourishment from food is to consume too much energy from food.

15. Sedentary people gain weight and fat as a means of staying healthy. Overweight is not normally a cause of illness. But obesity (not itself a disease) is associated with "Western" diseases of the alimentary tract (including the stomach and digestive system) and of the cardiovascular system (the heart, lungs and blood vessels). Processed "junk" food is a cause of obesity.

16. Some people eat much more processed food and sugars than others. People liable to suffer from deficiency states, or the "junk-food syndrome," include young office workers and housewives, youngsters, students, people living alone, heavy drinkers, anyone with a "sweet tooth," anyone who eats small amounts of fresh food, and dieters.

17. Dieters are liable to be in a state of acute malnutrition as a result of their dieting, unless they take care to eat only whole, fresh food, especially whole-meal bread and cereals. Most diets cut out such foods, and it is hard to avoid eating processed sugars, which are present in almost every type of manufactured food. Dieting can cause illness.

18. After a diet regime has ended, the body will signal acute hunger, in order to replace the nutrients of which it has been starved. This is the reason for the raging appetite and compulsive eating many dieters experience and is another reason why the body frustrates the dieter and becomes fatter after the diet. In Western countries, well-being often depends on being fat.

19. Processed sugars are worse than useless. As well as replacing nutritious foods, they drain the body of some vitamins and are a direct cause of various Western diseases. Eating sugar has the paradoxical effect of lowering the level of sugar in the blood. Processed sugars are a cause of diabetes, and heart disease, and are addictive. Eating sugar makes you hungry.

20. The body will always seek a level of energy balance at which the amount of nourishing food eaten will be sufficient for its needs. The body of anyone eating relatively little good food will therefore tend to slow down. Because people in the West eat a lot of food heavy in energy but poor in nourishment, they get heavier and fatter while eating less.

This is why people in Western countries tend to get fat. The next ten points summarize the means whereby we can lose fat and gain health.

21. A fire may burn bright with a small amount of good fuel and a gentle draft. With a strong draft a fire will burn faster and higher and use much fuel. As with a domestic fire, so with the human body. The more oxygen we breathe, the more food we will burn, and therefore the more nourishment we can consume. The fit body is the healthiest body.

22. Dieting slows the body down, lowering the metabolic rate as the body adjusts to less food. Exercise of the right type speeds the body up, raising the metabolic rate as the body needs more oxygen and therefore also more food. The effective type of exercise, which uses more oxygen, is "aerobic" exercise, sustained at a point just below breathlessness.

23. Aerobic exercise creates a sense of well-being which totally contrasts with the malaise of the junk-food syndrome. This is because the body of the aerobically fit person develops a hunger for the nourishing foods it needs: whole fresh foods in abundance, rich in protein, essential fats, fiber, vitamins and minerals, all vital to good health.

24. Western life has deprived us of the regular exercise and also of the nourishing food that was enjoyed by people who lived well before industrialization, and that is now enjoyed by settled communities who live away from Western influence. As a rule such people do not get fat and do not suffer from Western diseases. We have much to learn from them.

25. A couple of hours of aerobic exercise a week, divided into four sessions, will approximate the work that peasants do as a natural and necessary part of their lives. This exercise develops the muscle that uses fat as fuel and also strengthens the cardiovascular system. The result is a loss of fat, a gain of lean tissue, and a greatly reduced risk of Western diseases.

26. Grains (including wheat, corn, rice, oats), legumes (peas and beans) and tubers (especially potatoes) are the staple foods of non-Western societies, as they were in the West before industrialization. These foods are rich in starch, needed by the body and brain for energy, and also rich in protein, fiber, vitamins and minerals. They are truly the "staff of life."

27. Whole foods contain fiber, which exercises the alimentary tract. Food rich in fiber has an effect on the body which is totally opposite to that produced by processed sugars. Eating whole fresh food is a vital part of an active life, and will lead to a greatly reduced risk of diseases both of the cardiovascular system and of the alimentary tract.

28. Women have been taught to admire an ideal of slenderness, and to believe that dieting is the means to this end. Because dieting is self-defeating, it reinforces the sense of failure women often feel in a world run to suit men, and is damaging to women's mental as well as physical health. Women will gain self-respect by eating good food.

29. Women have also been taught to reject for themselves the ideals of strength, energy and competition, so women cling to dieting and resist exercise. It is time now for women to gain the freedom to enjoy their own bodies, to resist unreal stereotypes and to achieve energy, fitness and health by means of exercise that promotes a natural beauty.

30. Sedentary people who eat bad food usually get fat and then go on diets that do not work. The bad habits that lead to dieting also lead to disease. The body is nourished by good food and regenerated by exercise. These are the principal sources of good health. We become fit and healthy not by deprivation, but by using all our energies.

Index

About the Authors

GEOFFREY CANNON read Philosophy, Psychology and Physiology at Balliol College, Oxford, and was a founder member of the weekly journal *New Society*. After ten years at the BBC, as editor of *Radio Times,* he joined the *Sunday Times* in 1980 as an assistant editor. He has devised exercise programs for *Running* magazine, for which he writes a monthly column. Geoffrey Cannon is consultant editor of *New Health* magazine, and head of public affairs for the London Road Runners Club. His second book, *The Food Scandal,* cowritten with Caroline Walker, was published in 1984.

HETTY EINZIG is a free-lance journalist whose interest in women's health and related issues began while studying Modern Languages at Girton College, Cambridge. She has written for the *Sunday Times, Harpers & Queen* and various other publications.

YOUR BODY AND YOU

Do you know how much your body reveals about your thoughts, anxieties, personality? How important are the body's actions to mental well-being?

Find out with these popular books!

____62530	**DIETING MAKES YOU FAT** Geoffrey Cannon and Hetty Einzig	$3.95
____62012	**SUPERNUTRITION:** **MEGAVITAMIN REVOLUTION** Richard A. Passwater	$3.95
____54064	**BODYBUILDING FOR EVERYONE** Lou Ravelle	$3.50
____63418	**BODY LANGUAGE** Julius Fast	$3.95
____55462	**BODYBUILDING FOR WOMEN** Robert Kennedy	$3.50
____63600	**TOTAL FITNESS IN 30 MINUTES A WEEK** Laurence E. Morehouse, Ph.D. and Leonard Gross	$3.95
____53226	**LANGUAGE OF FEELINGS** David Viscott	$3.50
____46139	**ARNOLD: THE EDUCATION OF** **A BODYBUILDER** Arnold Schwartzenegger and Douglas Hall	$3.95

POCKET
BOOKS

HEALTH RELATED BOOKS YOU WILL WANT

____ THE COMPLETE BOOK OF ALLERGY CONTROL
      50886/$4.95
____ THE WAY OF HERBS
      46686/$4.95
____ COMPLETE VEGETARIAN COOKBOOK
      52642/$3.95
____ DR. MANDELL'S ALLERGY-FREE COOKBOOK
      49562/$3.50
____ DR. MANDELL'S 5-DAY ALLERGY RELIEF SYSTEM
      63061/$4.50
____ BACKACHE: STRESS AND TENSION
      50850/$2.95
____ CARLTON FREDERICKS' CALORIE AND
      CARBOHYDRATEE GUIDE 64274/$3.95
____ SUPERNUTRITION: MEGAVITAMIN
      REVOLUTION 62012/$3.95
____ HOW TO STOP SMOKING
      52460/$2.95
____ THE PRITIKIN PROMISE
      54634/$4.95
____ FREEDOM FROM BACKACHES
      62392/$3.95
____ FAMILY MEDICAL ENCYCLOPEDIA
      47794/$4.95
____ DLPA TO END CHRONIC PAIN
      AND DEPRESSION 63120/$7.95
____ THE NATURAL FOODS
      NUTRITION COUNTER 52845/$3.95

POCKET
BOOKS

Simon & Schuster, Mail Order Dept.   FHR
200 Old Tappan Rd., Old Tappan, N.J. 07675

Please send me the books I have checked above. I am enclosing $_____ (please add 75¢ to cover
postage and handling for each order. N.Y.S. and N.Y.C. residents please add appropriate sales tax). Send
check or money order—no cash or C.O.D.'s please. Allow up to six weeks for delivery. For purchases
over $10.00 you may use VISA: card number, expiration date and customer signature must be included.

Name _____

Address _____

City _____ State/Zip _____

VISA Card No. _____ Exp. Date _____

Signature _____
                                                              546